THE RESILIENT
WARRIOR

BEFORE, DURING, AND AFTER WAR

GLENN R. SCHIRALDI, PH.D.
LT. COLONEL, U.S. ARMY RESERVES (RETIRED)

RTI
Resilience Training International^SM
Ashburn, Virginia

Development of this booklet was made possible by a grant from **Rivers of Recovery,** a non-profit outdoor recreational/rehabilitation program for physically and psychologically injured veterans and active duty military service members and their families.

Rivers of Recovery
170 St. Moritz Strasse
Park City, UT 84098
Tel: 303-801-8022
www.riversofrecovery.org

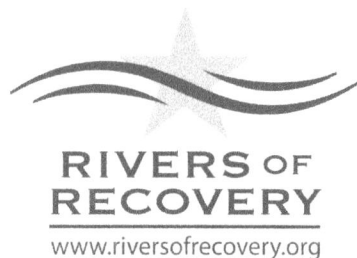

ISBN 978-0-9834755-0-7

Printed in the United States of America

Second printing 2012

Resilience Training International
20322 Bowfonds Street
Ashburn, VA 20147
www.resiliencefirst.com

Credits
Cover Design by Steve Palmer

This booklet may be found on www.Amazon.com

Praise for *The Resilient Warrior Before, During, and After War*

"A masterpiece! A definitive, complete, and absolutely essential guide to preparing for combat, surviving in combat, and after combat. "Required reading" for anyone in the military or law enforcement, for the families and loved ones of those who go in harm's way, and for those who treat or support the returning veteran. I truly am blown away by the depth of content and scholarship in this book. I believe that it should become the definitive reference source for anyone working in this field. Well done, my brother warrior-wordsmith and fellow warrior-healer! Hooah!"

> —Dave Grossman, Lt. Col. (Retired), Army Ranger, author *On Combat* and *On Killing*

"As a former small unit leader of Rangers, I wish I had this manuscript long ago. It is brilliantly conceived and well presented; a superb handbook with effective, poignant guidelines on avoiding the hurtful affects of PTSD and stress and how to deal with those problems. A must have booklet for all combatants and their families and friends."

> —Gary Dolan, Army Ranger, author *Of Their Own Accord*

"As a Navy SEAL wife who has been through a number of war zone deployments with my husband, I know how difficult homecoming can be for both people. I truly believe that this booklet will not only help normalize what so many people are experiencing when returning home from war zones but will also provide them, and their families, with tools to process the challenging events they have gone through. Very easy to read and understand…will reach people from all walks of life. Although my husband is honestly the most resilient, well-adjusted person I've ever known, this gives us much to talk about…a fantastic piece of work!"

> —Erin Roberts, wife of U.S. Navy SEAL

"A comprehensive handbook that provides an accessible and achievable roadmap to preparation, treatment, and recovery from the psychological stresses of combat. We are confident that this resource will prove invaluable to our participants."

> —Dan T. Cook, Founder, Executive Director, Rivers of Recovery

"This booklet should be read by all soldiers, especially leaders in the military. It will help them and those that serve with them to avoid PTSD and allow them to overcome post-traumatic stress without it becoming a disorder. I found the tools very useful and the steps easy to follow."

> —Kurt W. Roberts, Major, U.S. Army Infantry, OIF veteran

"This booklet has great utility, and I'm certain warfighters will respond to the analogies and calming techniques so eloquently described. I especially found the chapter on calming skills very insightful."

> —Sheila Galvin, FNP, Traumatic Brain Injury Program Coordinator, Wounded Warrior Regiment, USMC

"After reading Dr. Schiraldi's short, to-the-point, and easily digestible resource, I am convinced that our current generations of war fighters who may have returned from the fight "feeling just not right" have a great tool for success. The methods and processes within these pages hold the keys that will open the front doors to a mansion with many locked rooms. Practice and application will open the doors, allowing cross ventilation of the stifling air locked in the rooms, and helping to clear out the stale, pungent, dirty air that many are breathing each and every day. We can't change the past, but this booklet can affect the future. Best of luck to all readers! Semper Fidelis."

—John Ploskonka, Regimental Sergeant Major, USMC

"Glenn Schiraldi has once again offered much-needed education for stress syndromes—this time aimed directly at our service men and women. This guide is practical, easily read, and addresses the need for self-management skills before, during, and after deployment. Dr. Schiraldi's devotion to our military members, families, and communities is evident in this book."

—Victoria Bruner, LCSW, RN, BCETS, Associate Director of Clinical Education, Deployment Health Clinical Center, Walter Reed Army Medical Center

"Dr. Glenn Schiraldi has offered a timely, insightful perspective on stress management for soldiers and their families, especially those of the post-9/11 generation. No generation has been asked to do more for our great Nation, and none has responded more superbly. Dr. Schiraldi honors their service by providing clear explanations of the stress they confront and concise suggestions on how to maintain resilience in their professional and personal lives."

—Robert M. Kimmitt, Major General, USAR (Retired), 173rd Airborne Brigade, Vietnam, 1970-71

These comments reflect the views of the individuals only, and not those of any U.S. government agency.

Introduction

War changes everyone. Many of these changes are for the good, and some can be very challenging to live with. This booklet will be useful if you are a military service member—active duty or veteran—who has served or is preparing to serve in a war zone. It will also be helpful for government workers or contractors who deploy, and for the families of those who deploy.

This booklet is about building resilience. Resilience helps warriors handle the strains of life—especially military life. As you improve your resilience skills, you'll probably feel better, perform better, and enjoy yourself more.

Don't worry about remembering everything in this booklet. Just try to learn as much as you can, and keep the booklet as a ready reference. You'll likely find all the principles and skills in this booklet helpful at one time or another. However, everyone is different. If you have questions or concerns, be sure to write them down (there's space for notes at the back), and ask your doctor or other helping professional about them before you try a new skill. Add any of your own notes that may help you later. Please be aware that this booklet is intended to augment proper medical or psychological care, not replace it.

What Is Resilience?

Resilience is those strengths of mind and character—both inborn and developed—that help us to respond well to adversity. The strengths of resilience help us to:

- Perform at our very best, even under pressure
- Prevent and recover from combat stress-related problems, such as post-traumatic stress disorder, depression, anxiety, problem anger, drug/substance abuse, and difficulty connecting with others
- Maintain and improve peak mental fitness throughout life

Who Is Resilient?

You are, or you wouldn't have made it this far. Congratulations for surviving very difficult times. Yet just as a world-class athlete constantly works at improving his game, so can you enhance your resilience at any time in your life. This booklet will help you build upon your strengths. Everyone can move up the staircase of resilience, starting where you are now. You are more fortunate than many in that you are already beginning the process of building resilience.

Why Is Resilience So Important?

Resilience helps us to be our best mentally, physically, emotionally, socially, and functionally. This might be all the motivation you need to build your resilience. However, ten to forty percent of people return from deployment with troubling symptoms related to combat stress. These symptoms might go away with time. Often they don't—or get worse. These symptoms can interfere with your ability to work, be happy, and be fully there for your buddies or loved ones. Resilience training will help you recognize these symptoms and quickly apply new skills to lessen them. When additional help is needed, resilience training will also help you get the right assistance so that you can return to your best. Finally, resilience skills might help to prevent one with combat stress symptoms from becoming a combat-stress casualty.

You are probably well trained in the tactics of war. This booklet will give you the tools to take excellent care of yourself. Once you get good at these skills, you'll become a resource to help others you care about become more resilient.

What Can I Expect?

Practicing the principles and skills in this booklet, then, will help you to:
- Reduce the excessive arousal of stress that interferes with health and performance
- Manage strong negative emotions and stress symptoms
- Recover from combat stress and trauma
- Prevent certain stress-related disorders and/or relapse
- Thrive and be stronger
- Optimize mental health and functioning on the job and at home or garrison
- Improve physical health (The mind and body are connected. Unmanaged stress symptoms can lead to serious medical conditions, ranging from headaches to chronic pain, sleep disruptions, obesity, diabetes, drug abuse, high blood pressure, and heart disease.)
- Enjoy life more, thus increasing career retention (Those who are happy tend to stay at their jobs longer.)
- Become a resource for others

Contents

The booklet is organized into the following chapters:

One

About Combat Stress

If you know neither yourself nor your enemy, you will always endanger yourself.

Sun Tzu, *The Art of War*

The warrior defends those who can't defend themselves, by protecting their physical safety, their liberty, and their highest ideals. The warrior's life is one of service, sacrifice, and often hardship. As a warrior, you well understand the price of preserving liberty.

War is a double-edged sword. War zone experience exposes you to some of life's best, such as:

- Meeting some of the finest people, and establishing strong bonds and friendships
- Witnessing acts of courage, selflessness, honor, and skill
- Feeling justified pride in enduring more adversity than most, overcoming challenges, and facing your fears and other strong emotions
- Becoming aware of, and appreciating, your strengths and capacities
- Gaining more wisdom, maturity, discipline, self-confidence, and self-reliance
- Knowing that you can endure hardship and bounce back from a wide range of emotions
- Having a greater appreciation for liberty, life, peace, love, family, and other things that matter most in life
- Finding a greater sense of meaning and purpose
- Cultivating a greater appreciation of simple pleasures and quiet moments
- Feeling self-satisfaction from doing your best in difficult times and standing up to injustice
- Having opportunities for leadership, teamwork, career, education, adventure, and travel
- Experiencing spiritual growth

Adversity can indeed enrich life. However, war can also involve loss and pain, such as:

- Separation from loved ones (and sometimes loss of relationships)
- Killing
- Seeing killing and death
- Physical injury to self or others
- Awareness of your limits and shortcomings (Although this can eventually lead to wisdom and growth, it might also cause guilt, sadness, anger, and anxiety.)
- Disappointment in the weaknesses and mistakes of others
- Loss of innocence—realizing that people can be bad, that good doesn't always prevail, that women and children can't always be trusted; feeling changed and different from those who haven't served in a war zone
- Difficulty managing strong, expected emotions like grief, sadness, fear, guilt, rage, and helplessness (e.g., from IEDs, restrictive rules of engagement, snipers, watching buddies die)

So be open to the gains from war zone experience, while accepting and preparing for its unique challenges.

Combat Stress Reactions

When we face a dangerous situation, the brain orchestrates a number of changes called the stress response, or just stress, which prepare us for fight or flight. Normally stress helps us to function better. When combat stress is extreme or prolonged, however, a number of changes can degrade performance. These changes range from relatively mild (e.g., fatigue, dizziness, feeling jumpy) to severe (e.g., total exhaustion, inability to move, vacant stare, trembling, hyperventilation, insomnia, indecisiveness, loss of confidence, carelessness, frequent crying, inability to relax, unusually strong anger). These are all normal. Even severe reactions usually respond favorably to a few days of rest, reassurance, and use of the skills explained in this booklet.

Post-Traumatic Stress Disorder

Many warriors return from deployment with symptoms of post-traumatic stress disorder (PTSD). A few things are important to know about PTSD. First, nearly all of the symptoms of PTSD are normal reactions for a warrior in combat. Indeed, they might be considered essential for survival. Thus, expect that in a war zone you will be "wired"—physically aroused and ready to fight, highly alert to danger and changes in your surroundings, remembering battles and their lessons, etc. Second, you can have some symptoms of PTSD without having PTSD. In fact, it is likely that you'll experience at least some symptoms after serving in a war zone. Third, if you carry unresolved traumatic memories from earlier in your life into combat, you might be more likely to develop PTSD. Thus, it is wise to make sure that troubling memories of sexual trauma, abuse of any kind, or especially distressing military experiences are settled before you face new potentially traumatic experiences. Assistance from professionals can help when your own efforts don't. (More about this later.) Fourth, while PTSD might be considered a normal response to an abnormal situation (like combat, rape, or domestic violence), problems occur when the symptoms become extreme and persistent. For example, some anger might help you to focus and persist in combat. However, if months after returning from the war zone, anger festers, you fly off the handle at small things (e.g., someone moves your stuff, acts irresponsibly, or doesn't stay in communication with you), you throw things, or you are hurting yourself or others verbally or physically, this is *not* normal. Combat turns on the normal stress response. In PTSD, the stress response doesn't turn off. Finally, PTSD rarely occurs alone. Depression, anxiety/panic attacks, substance use disorder, and other symptoms of excessive stress usually occur along with PTSD as people try to deal with unresolved traumatic memories that they weren't prepared for.

Many of the skills in this booklet will help you to turn down the symptoms of PTSD when you don't need to be on high alert. If symptoms persist, get worse, and/or are troubling (e.g., interfering with your happiness, relationships, or ability to do what you want to do), pay attention. PTSD is highly treatable, even in combat vets, if you access the full range of treatments that are available. Once you can acknowledge your own PTSD symptoms and learn how to recover from them, you can better help others. For example, you can tell people that treatment does help, that they don't have to suffer needlessly for years, that they can return to a "new normal," and be 100% there for their buddies and loved ones again.

If you have had a concussion (also called mild traumatic brain injury), lingering symptoms are far more likely to be caused by PTSD than the concussion (99% of brain injuries in warriors are concussions, which usually heal with time and rest).

For self-awareness, you might try completing the PTSD checklist on the next page. Knowing what to look for will benefit yourself and others. When you finish, check the scoring information that follows the checklist.

PTSD Symptoms Checklist—Military Version*

The following is a list of problems or complaints that can occur after one has been in a war zone. Circle the numbers to indicate how much each symptom has bothered you in the last month.

Symptom	(1) Not at all	(2) A little bit	(3) Moderately	(4) Quite a bit	(5) Extremely
1. Repeated, disturbing memories, thoughts, or images of a stressful military experience.	1	2	3	4	5
2. Repeated, disturbing dreams of a stressful military experience.	1	2	3	4	5
3. Suddenly acting or feeling as if a stressful military experience were happening again (as if you were reliving it).	1	2	3	4	5
4. Feeling very upset when something reminded you of a stressful military experience.	1	2	3	4	5
5. Having physical reactions (e.g., heart pounding, trouble breathing, or sweating) when something reminded you of a stressful military experience.	1	2	3	4	5
6. Avoid thinking about or talking about a stressful military experience, or avoid having feelings related to it.	1	2	3	4	5
7. Avoid activities or situations because they remind you of a stressful military experience.	1	2	3	4	5
8. Trouble remembering important parts of a stressful military experience.	1	2	3	4	5
9. Loss of interest in things that you used to enjoy; you don't seem to care.	1	2	3	4	5
10 Feeling distant or cut off from other people.	1	2	3	4	5
11. Feeling emotionally numb or being unable to have loving feelings for those close to you.	1	2	3	4	5
12. Feeling as if your future will somehow be cut short or not be normal.	1	2	3	4	5
13. Trouble falling or staying asleep.	1	2	3	4	5
14. Feeling irritable or having angry outbursts.	1	2	3	4	5
15. Having difficulty concentrating.	1	2	3	4	5
16. Being "super alert" or watchful, on guard.	1	2	3	4	5
17. Feeling jumpy or easily startled.	1	2	3	4	5

*Slightly adapted from the PCL-M by Weathers, Litz, Huska, and Keane of the National Center for PTSD. Note that PTSD can also result from experiencing or witnessing dangerous situations such as rape, terrorism, abuse (sexual, physical, perhaps even verbal), torture, car accidents, or natural disasters.

Scoring

Total the score by adding the seventeen circled numbers. A total score of less than 30 is considered low symptoms ("normal"), 30-39 indicates some symptoms, 40-49 moderate symptoms, and 50 or more is considered high symptoms of PTSD. Pay particular attention to items whose score is 3 or more. Scores of 40 or greater usually suggest the need for professional evaluation/assistance. However, the total score is just one estimate of PTSD. It is also important to consider how much suffering symptoms cause, and how much they interfere with your happiness or ability to do what you want (at home, your job, relationships, recreation, and so on).

Let's begin now to learn the principles and skills of resilience. Whether your goal is to improve performance, optimize mental fitness, prevent stress-related disorders, or recover from excessive distress, resilience will help you accomplish your goals.

Two

The Resilient Brain

Resilience starts with the brain. The resilient brain enables you to learn, remember, size up problems, make and execute decisions, follow instructions, and regulate moods—and does all of this fairly quickly. We now know that there is much you can do to attain and maintain sharp brain functioning. As you consider how much the condition of the brain affects your success, you'll likely care for your brain as well as you do your body and your equipment. This chapter is about peak brain health and functioning. If you think of your brain as a computer, then this chapter will focus on strengthening the "hardware," while future chapters will focus on the "software," or learning.

The brain consists of 100 billion neurons, or nerve cells. Each neuron connects and communicates with thousands of others. In consistency, the brain is like Jello, suggesting the importance of protecting the head. Three regions, shown in the figure below, are particularly critical to peak brain functioning:

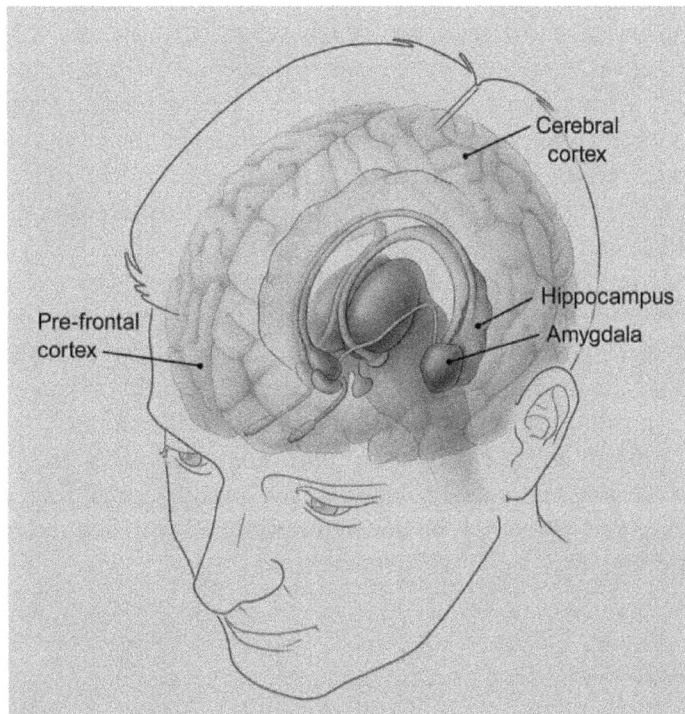

©2004 Haderer & Müller Biomedical Art, LLC. Reprinted with permission.

1. **The pre-frontal cortex** (PFC) sits behind the forehead. If the brain is the command post of the body, then the PFC is the commander. The PFC considers what is going on all around, considers facts and memories that are stored elsewhere in the brain, and then plans, decides, initiates action, and regulates emotions. The PFC considers emotions until a decision feels right—when facts and feelings come together. Emotional input comes from the next two structures.
2. **The amygdala** picks up cues from the environment (especially dangerous ones), alerts the brain to feelings, and trips an emotional reaction and the stress response without conscious thought. So the amygdala informs the PFC of feelings, and allows us to feel strong emotions and their associated bodily sensations. If the amygdala were acting alone, we might jump or run from a fearful situation only to think about it later. But the amygdala doesn't act alone.

3. **The hippocampus** sits next to the amygdala and balances it. While the amygdala deals in strong emotions and promotes quick and unthinking reactions, the hippocampus deals in cold facts and promotes cool, rational thought. In effect, the hippocampus tells the PFC, "Let's consider all the facts before jumping." The hippocampus calmly calls up relevant memories that are stored elsewhere and feeds them to the PFC. So now the PFC allows you to think, "OK, the enemy is near, but we've trained well and we've performed well in similar situations before."

When the dangerous situation is over, the hippocampus stores what you've experienced in memory, in a rather cool, rational way. The amygdala gives emotions to the stored memories. In the healthy brain all three structures act in balance. You want to be alert to feelings, but too much uncontrolled feelings can get us into trouble. The PFC and the hippocampus temper the strong emotions of the amygdala.

When Things Go Wrong

Two factors can upset this delicate balance: excessive stress and aging. The stress hormone named *cortisol* sharpens thinking in the short term. However, when stress is excessive or prolonged, cortisol begins to disrupt brain function in several ways: Cortisol over-activates the amygdala. This can lead to excessive anxiety or other strong, negative emotions that hinder learning and cool action. The over-active amygdala also imprints memories with excessive, intense emotions, which is what happens in PTSD. In addition, cortisol shrinks and/or disrupts the hippocampus and PFC. These two structures are vital to straight thinking and keeping the amygdala calm. In a similar way, aging can cause shrinkage and/or disruption in the PFC and hippocampus.

But there is good news. We have learned in recent years that the brain is plastic. That is, neurons that are destroyed by cortisol can regrow, the connections between neurons can be strengthened, and the strength and functioning of neurons can improve as we exercise, eat well, rest, learn new coping skills, and practice the other steps you'll learn in this chapter.

We have also learned that brain health equals heart health. What affects the heart also affects the brain. Thus, it is important to: (1) stay lean, particularly around the abdomen, (2) keep blood pressure, blood sugar, blood fats, and total cholesterol low, and (3) keep good cholesterol (HDL) high.

Research is showing that much can be done to optimize brain health and function. Let's discuss what you need to know to develop a more resilient brain.

Regular Exercise

Exercise—particularly aerobic exercise—tunes up the brain hardware in many ways, priming it to learn. Exercise produces master molecules in the brain that normally decrease with stress and aging. These molecules stimulate the growth of neurons and supportive tissue, protect neurons from deterioration, promote the transmission of signals between neurons, and improve blood and oxygen flow to the brain by growing new blood vessels. Exercise increases brain volume overall, particularly in the PFC and hippocampus. It is well established that exercise is associated with better performance, mood, and heart health, and less fatigue, joint problems, anxiety, depression, and obesity. Exercise also lowers high cortisol levels, which can damage neurons.

Build up gradually and don't push too quickly so as to avoid discouragement. Strive for aerobic exercise all or nearly all days. To your aerobic base, try adding strength training, flexibility training, and complex movements (such as marital arts, ping pong, juggling, yoga, tai chi, dancing, or playing a musical instrument) to further sharpen brain function. Learning something new causes the brain to forge new neural pathways that improve brain functioning. Outdoor exercise is good—ten to fifteen minutes of sunlight a few times a week raises levels of vitamin D, which improves brain function.

Sleep

Sleep is necessary to energize and refresh the brain. People generally do not appreciate how even a little sleep deprivation seriously affects mood and performance. Most adults require about eight hours of sleep per night to feel and function at their best. Anything less than seven to eight hours of sleep per night will degrade performance, and usually mood. Military researchers have found that sleep shortage quickly and significantly impairs the ability to remember, make decisions, and perform tasks requiring speed and accuracy. Think, for example, of having to fire at a pop-up target compared to a stationary one. Even losing two hours of sleep results in *many* more mental errors. Sleep shortage seems to impair the hippocampus, blocking our ability to problem-solve and settle traumatic memories. Like stress, sleep shortage also raises cortisol, and increases the risks of weight gain, high blood pressure, and a number of other medical diseases. So think of sleep discipline as effective human resource management.

Two principles are critical: *amount* and *regularity*. Strive for 7-8 hours of sleep each day. Try to vary times for going to sleep and awakening by no more than one hour per night to help the brain regulate sleep cycles—even on the weekends. Napping partially offsets sleep loss. Nap in a quiet, dark place for thirty minutes or longer if you can (eye shades and ear plugs can help). When it's time to sleep, turn off the digital/electronic devices and go to bed. Instead of using these to relax, wind down with music, reading, journal writing, prayer, or a relaxation technique (see chapter 3). Realize that light, even from a computer screen, and noise can interfere with sleep, even when you don't think they do. As much as possible, shut down light sources an hour before going to bed, block out light and noise, and/or try white noise, eye shades, or ear plugs.

Exercise generally aids sleep. Early-morning exercise helps to regulate sleep rhythms. Tai chi and yoga usually help, as well. Try to avoid exercising within two hours of bedtime.

Don't eat a heavy meal or drink excessive fluid before bedtime. Try a lighter meal a few hours before going to bed, and have a light snack before bedtime, such as warm low- or no-fat milk and honey. Milk's tryptophan promotes sleep (the carbohydrate in honey helps the tryptophan enter the brain), and the protein might prevent your awakening from low blood sugar. Other good snacks are yogurt, a banana, walnuts, almonds, an egg, avocado, tuna, turkey, oatmeal, or a cup of cereal and milk. Caffeine, nicotine, and alcohol interfere with sleep, especially if taken in the hours before bedtime.

Brain-Healthy Nutrition

In focusing on weight loss, we often forget that nutrients from food are critical to optimal brain health, functioning, and mood. The so-called power, or functional, foods—plants (vegetables, fruits, legumes, nuts, and whole grains) and fish—greatly benefit the brain. It is also good to limit high-fat dairy products, red meat, sugar, and salt. Fortunately, the rules of heart-healthy eating apply to brain-healthy eating, so we'll briefly underscore the principles. If you think of a plate full of plant foods, with meat as a small side dish, you'll likely get most of these principles.

1. *Choose good carbohydrates.* The brain functions best with a steady supply of blood sugar (glucose). Low-carbohydrate diets work against good brain function by depleting stores of glucose. On the other hand, spikes in blood sugar are not brain friendly. Nature packages unprocessed plant products (*whole* grains, fresh or frozen vegetables and fruits, nuts, beans, and so on) with fiber, which slows the absorption of sugar into the blood, and antioxidants, which promote neuron health. Conversely, refined carbohydrates lack antioxidants, fiber, and other brain-friendly nutrients, and give spikes in blood sugar. Refined foods include those made with white flour and sugar (e.g., sodas with sugar or high fructose corn syrup, candy, cake, many cereals, white rice, pasta). Even a few sugary sodas a day instead of water appears to impair

brain health and function, while upping the risk for weight gain and several diseases. Look for whole grain products, which will also help you stay lean—such as brown rice, whole wheat, oats of any kind, and so forth.

2. *Maximize the intake of antioxidants.* Antioxidants reduce the damage to neurons caused by stress and aging, raise HDL, and sharpen brain function. Antioxidants are found in colorful plant foods. These include red grapes, blueberries, strawberries, tomatoes, broccoli, spinach, apples, chocolate (yes, a little each day is good), green or black tea, oranges, and cantaloupe. Antioxidants are even found in pale plants, such as pears, white beans, green grapes, cauliflower, and soybeans. Antioxidants are also plentiful in spices (cinnamon, cloves, oregano, allspice, marjoram, rosemary, sage, tarragon, thyme, cumin, saffron, fennel, garlic, basil, ginger, pepper, turmeric) if stored in a cool, dark, place and consumed within two years. Don't forget the antioxidants found in the germ and bran of whole grain products and in nuts.

3. *Eat enough but not too much.* Try to stop eating before you are full, as long-living populations do. Studies indicate that this benefits the brain.

4. *Aim to eat at least 2-3 servings of fish per week, totaling at least eight ounces.* The omega-3 fatty acids in fish (called DHA and EPA) are critical components of the neurons in the brain. These fatty-acids improve brain function and health, mood, and heart health, while reducing depression and possibly reducing stress in traumatized people. Avoid fried fish, as frying adds unhealthy fats, which cancel omega-3's benefits. To reduce the risk of contaminants, choose wild fish as much as possible, and remove the skin. If you choose to use fish oil supplements, look to consume 500-1000 mg of DHA and EPA (as opposed to total mg of fish oil) daily.

5. *Choose good fats.* In combination with sugar, saturated animal fats damage neurons. So minimize cheeseburgers and other fatty meats, French fries, shakes, full-fat dairy products, pies, and super-sized sodas. Trans-fats, found in processed, fast, and restaurant foods, are worse. Replace unhealthy fats with fats from plants (nuts, avocados, olive oil, canola oil, peanut oil) and use low- or no-fat dairy products (which actually appear to promote heart health).

6. *Consider vitamin supplements.* No pill will make up for an unhealthy diet. However, many researchers think that sufficient vitamin D is linked to better mental function. Ten to fifteen minutes of sunlight on the skin toward mid-day or up to 1000 IU of vitamin D3 in supplement form can be helpful. Some research suggests that B vitamins might also improve mood and functioning. A good quality multivitamin supplement will provide about 100% of needed daily amounts.

7. *Hydrate.* Even a 2% weight loss from perspiration can affect mental and physical functioning and mood (this would be a loss of four pounds in water weight for a 200-pound person). Assuming normal eating, you will likely need to drink around 9 to 13 cups of liquid per day— more if you are large in size or active, even in cooler climates. Drink liquid before you are thirsty and often (every 15-20 minutes). You can see if you are getting enough fluid by checking the color of your urine. It should look like pale lemonade (or Bud Light), when you look at the urine stream, a cup of urine (the first void of the day is the best measure), or the urine that settles in the toilet bowl. If the urine is darker, increase your fluid intake.

8. *Eat a good breakfast.* Studies consistently show that breakfast eaters are leaner and perform better. Protein prolongs the sense of fullness throughout the day. Good protein sources are low- or no-fat milk or yogurt, egg whites, poultry, seafood, beans, nuts, peanut butter, and protein powder. Replace foods that give rapid sugar spikes (like bagels, white bread, pastries, processed cereals, English muffins, pancakes, or waffles) with oatmeal, barley, or other whole-grain cereals, whole wheat bread, and fresh or frozen fruit.

9. *Reduce salt.* Most salt comes from processed foods.

Think more about eating what you need, rather than what you should avoid. Most nutrition experts agree that eating more vegetables and fruits is the number one nutritional priority for Americans. The average adult should get five servings of vegetables (which can include beans) and four servings of fruits. Most get far fewer. Again think of filling your plate up with plant-based foods. The average adult will also need 3 cups of low- or no-fat dairy.

Substances

Brain imaging can detect abnormalities in brain function caused by substances years before structural damage is apparent. Brain imaging teaches us to avoid the following, all of which degrade the structure and function of the brain:

- *Alcohol in excess*. Most who drink exceed the recommended daily upper limit of one drink for women and two for men. Four to five drinks a day, even occasionally, is particularly risky.
- *Smoking*. Smoking tobacco greatly increases the risk of depression and anxiety. Pot smoking is also harmful.
- *Caffeine in excess*. Three cups of coffee a day appear safe.
- *Any other "recreational" or illicit drug.*

The figure below shows the effects of substances on brain function, as measured by nuclear brain imaging. A healthy, well-functioning brain appears smooth, as on the two center scans.

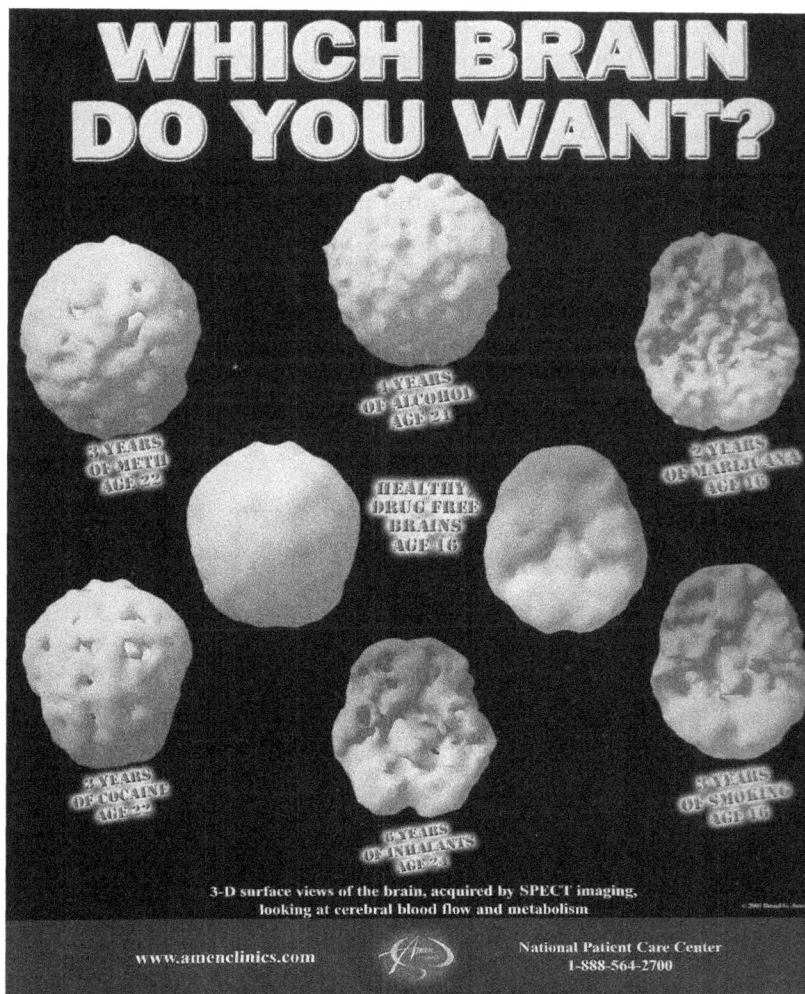

Reprinted by permission of Dr. Daniel Amen. www.AmenClinics.com. ©2005 Daniel G. Amen.

Any drug, in excess, increases the harmful scalloping effects seen around the perimeter of the figure. Starting at the top and going clockwise, these scans reflect excesses in alcohol, marijuana, smoking, inhalants, cocaine, and methamphetamine.

Medical conditions

Sleep apnea interferes with restful sleep and can leave one feeling mentally sluggish, tired, and depressed. It can cause insomnia, headaches, nightmares, high blood pressure, strokes, and heart attacks. Apnea is common in people with PTSD; treating apnea often lessens nightmares and other PTSD symptoms. Loud snoring, stoppage of breathing, and loud gasps for air as people partially awaken to breathe signal apnea. Apnea is very effectively treated. Ask your doctor about this. Losing 5-10 pounds of weight might help, as does limiting alcohol, sedatives, sleeping pills, and muscle relaxants.

Also check for and treat the following, which all affect brain health: elevated cholesterol (which can sometimes cause depression); thyroid disorders (ask for a TSH test to rule out problems that might cause anxiety, depression, mental sluggishness, sleep problems, elevated cholesterol, and many other unexplained problems); high blood pressure (reducing sodium/salt intake helps, as does increasing plant foods); diabetes; and gum disease (brush and floss daily to prevent toxins from entering the bloodstream and avoid tobacco).

Many medications interfere with the transmission of messages between neurons in the brain. These include antihistamines, tranquilizers (such as benzodiazepines), sleeping pills, Tagamet, Zantac, and tricyclic antidepressants. Try to take such medications only as long as needed, or ask about trying other medications or treatments. For example, the newer selective serotonin reuptake inhibitors used for depression actually seem to strengthen the hippocampus, while other treatments for depression, such as cognitive therapy, are as effective as tricyclic antidepressants.

Finally, sunlight or sitting in front of a light box that approximates sunlight for 30-60 minutes daily has been found to improve depression and might improve mental performance.

Managing stress helps to reduce stress hormones that harm the brain and promote weight gain. The skills that we'll explore now will help you handle stress confidently.

Three

Calming Skills

Some stress is good. Excessive stress arousal (hereafter called *arousal*) is not. Excessive arousal is common to PTSD, anxiety, panic attacks, depression, substance use disorders, and problem anger. Excessive arousal also rapidly degrades performance in many ways. For example, when heart rate exceeds 145 beats per minute, warriors can experience loss of coordination, shaking voice, vision and hearing problems, deterioration in decision-making and judgment, and freezing, followed by memory loss, exhaustion, and nausea afterwards. So calming skills are essential survival skills. Excessive arousal is manifested *physically* (rapid and shallow breathing, racing or erratic heart rate, tight muscles, heavy perspiration), *emotionally* (overly reactive, excessively strong negative emotions), and *mentally* (negative thoughts, worry, difficulty concentrating, poor decision making).

The mind and body are connected, so you can start by calming the body, and the mind follows. Or, you can calm the mind, and the body follows. We'll begin with calming the body. Aerobic exercise is a good starting point. Now you'll add skills that will help you calm down when you get overly aroused—as everyone does from time to time—so that you can feel and function at your best. Practice these skills so that you can use them under pressure, or afterwards to calm stress symptoms.

Calm (Tactical) Breathing

For centuries, warriors have used breath awareness and control to calm down. Even small shifts in the rate or way we breathe can have profound affects on our state of mind and functioning—including headaches, unreal feelings, panic attacks, unsteadiness, and all the other symptoms of excessive arousal. As breathing calms, the ability to think, remember, and perform improves. Try this skill:
1. Sit in the meditator's posture, with feet flat on the floor, hands not touching and resting in your lap, and your back comfortably erect, supported by the back of a chair. Notice your level of stress.
2. Now take a moment to consciously relax the muscles of your mouth, jaw, throat, shoulders, chest, and abdomen. Place one hand over your navel, and the other over your breastbone. Breathe in through your nose so that only your lower hand moves, as if your abdomen were inflating. As you breathe out the hand falls. The upper body remains relaxed and still. The breathing is quiet and relaxed, without any gasps or holding of the breath. Breathe this way for thirty seconds. Notice how you feel.
3. Practice this often so that when you are distressed you will almost automatically relax your muscles and breathe abdominally.

Lt. Colonel Dave Grossman teaches a variation that warriors often use to perform better under pressure or distress. Simply relax your muscles as before. Breathe in slowly through the nose for the count of four, expanding your belly. Hold the breath for the count of four, breathe out through the lips for the count of four, and then hold for the count of four. Repeat this up to three times.

Experiment to see which type of breathing works best for you. The key is to practice so that you will call up this skill when you most need it.

Progressive Muscle Relaxation (PMR)

It has been demonstrated that when people relax their muscles they become mentally calmer. However, most people are not good at consciously relaxing. Paradoxically, first tensing the muscles actually helps the brain to more deeply relax the body. Like calm breathing, PMR is effective for nearly everyone fairly quickly. Daily practice lowers baseline arousal, but you can also use this to help you sleep and to calm down under pressure.

In PMR, you first tense, then relax different muscle groups. Pay attention first to the feeling of tension, and then to its opposite, relaxation. Concentrating on the difference helps retrain the brain to detect muscle tension as it first arises and reduce it. When you relax, muscles get longer and warmer as blood flow increases. You'll notice this sensation.

Read through the instructions below, and then try them. (Or, you might wish to audio-record these instructions or have someone else read them to you.) Prepare by getting comfortable—lie down on your back, remove glasses, loosen tight belts or collars, and so forth. You can also do this sitting down, with obvious adjustments to the instructions. You'll tense each muscle group for about 5-10 seconds, stopping short of discomfort, then relax for at least that long.

Begin by closing your eyes and breathe calmly and abdominally for a few seconds. As your breathing settles, begin PMR.

1. Point both of your feet and toes away from the head at the same time, leaving the legs relaxed. Notice tension in the calves and bottom of the feet. Relax and notice the contrast in those areas.
2. Bend the feet at the ankles so that the toes move toward your head. Sense the tension in the muscles below the knee, along the outside of the shins. Relax and notice the difference.

Continue this pattern of tensing…noticing…relaxing…noticing, as follows:

3. Tense the quadriceps on the front of your upper leg by straightening your legs and locking your knees. Leave your feet relaxed.
4. Tense the back of your legs by pressing the back of your heels against the floor or bed, as if you were lying on your back and digging your heels into the sand on a beach. Keep the toes pointing skyward. Sense tension along the entire back of the legs.
5. Squeeze the buttocks or seat muscles together while contracting your pelvic muscles.
6. Tense your stomach muscles by pulling them inward. Notice how a tight gut impedes breathing.
7. Tense your back muscles along both sides of the spine by slowly arching your back, pulling your chest up and toward the chin, while leaving your shoulders and buttocks down on the surface.
8. Shrug your shoulders, noticing tension above the collarbones and between the shoulder blades.
9. Tense the muscles in the top of the forearms. With palms down on the surface beside your body, pull the relaxed hands back at the wrists, with fingers pointing upward.
10. Tighten the fists and biceps, drawing the hands to the shoulders, as if lifting weights (curls). Notice tension in the fists, forearms, and biceps.
11. Very, very slowly rotate the chin to the right as if looking over your right shoulder, noticing tension along the right side of the neck. Slowly return to center, and then rotate to the left.
12. Press the head back gently against the surface you are lying on, while raising the chin toward the ceiling. Sense tension at the base of the skull, where it meets the neck.
13. Lift your eyebrows up and furrow your brow, sensing tension across the forehead.
14. Frown, pulling the corners of the mouth down—sensing tension on the sides of the chin and neck.
15. Grit your teeth and sense tension from the angle of the jaw up to the temple.
16. Grin ear to ear and sense tension around the cheekbones.

Spend a few more moments just resting and relaxing before going to sleep or getting up.

Heart Coherence

Thanks to new computer technology, we now know that calming the heart powerfully affects the mind, performance, and the rest of the body. The heart communicates to the brain and the rest of the body via nerves, hormones, blood pressure, and electromagnetic messages. In fact, there is much more messaging from the heart to the brain than from the brain to the heart. So regulating the heart is a powerful skill.

Generally, a lower heart rate favors health and performance. However, the *patterns* of the heart rhythms are even more important. It is possible to record beat-to-beat changes in heart rate. *Heart coherence* reflects the heart's ability to adjust speeds smoothly, flexibly, and quickly. Notice the figure below,[i] which shows a coherent heart on the left and a struggling heart on the right. Although both hearts have the same average resting heart rate (in beats per minute), the pattern on the left shows a balance between the two branches of the nervous system responsible for increasing and decreasing arousal. The coherent heart speeds up and slows down with easy regularity, like a world-class athlete who accelerates and slows down smoothly as the situation requires.

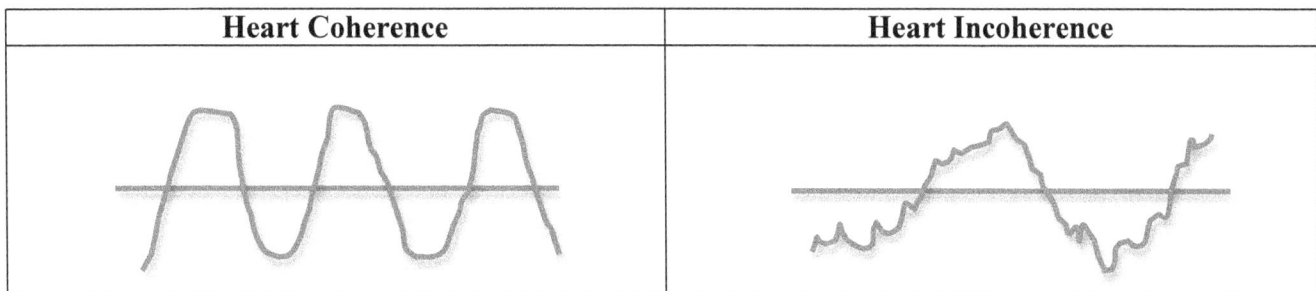

Heart Coherence	Heart Incoherence

Through practice, one can learn to achieve heart coherence in a matter of weeks or months. Research has established many benefits of heart coherence, including *mental* (less depression, anxiety, PTSD, anger, and stress; greater sense of well-being), *physical* (lower blood pressure; less pain, fatigue, and sleeplessness; lower cholesterol, cortisol, and weight levels), and *functional* (improved productivity, concentration, thinking, and listening ability).

Since emotions are experienced in the body, not the head (e.g., "my heart is down"; "I'm broken hearted"; "heart-felt appreciation"), it is effective to start at the heart level. The general principle is that any positive emotion experienced in the heart tends to elicit heart coherence.

The basic heart coherence technique, called The Quick Coherence® Technique,[ii] takes only a minute, but has powerful effects. Here are the instructions:

1. *Heart focus*. Focus your attention in the area of your heart. If this sounds confusing, try this: Focus on our right big toe and wiggle it. Now focus on your right elbow. Now gently focus in the center of your chest, the area of your heart. (Most people think the heart is on the left side of the chest, but it's really closer to the center, behind the breastbone.) If you like, you can put your hand over your heart to help. If your mind wanders, just keep shifting your attention back to the area of your heart. Now you're ready for the next step, Heart Breathing.
2. *Heart Breathing*. As you focus on the area of your heart, imagine your breath is flowing in and out through that area. This helps your mind and energy to stay focused in the heart area and your respiration and heart rhythms to synchronize. Breathe slowly and gently in through your heart (to a count of five or six) and slowly and easily out through your heart (to a count of five

---

[i] Adapted with permission from Childre, D., & Rozman, D. (2003). *Transformng Anger: The HeartMath Solution for Letting Go of Rage, Frustration, and Irritation.* Oakland, CA: New Harbinger, p. 21. ©2003 D. Childre & D. Rozman. Not to be reproduced without written permission.

[ii] Reprinted with permission from Childre, D., & Rozman, D. (2005). *Transforming Stress: The HeartMath Solution for Relieving Worry, Fatigue, and Tension.* Oakland, CA: New Harbinger, pp. 44-45. ©2005 by D. Childre and D. Rozman. Not to be reproduced without written permission.

or six). Do this until your breathing feels smooth and balanced, not forced. You may discover that it's easier to find a slow and easy rhythm by counting "one thousand, two thousand," rather than "one, two." Continue to breathe with ease until you find a natural inner rhythm that feels good to you.

3. *Heart feeling*. Continue to breathe through the area of your heart. As you do so, recall a positive feeling, a time when you felt good inside, and try to re-experience it. This could be a feeling of appreciation or care toward a special person or a pet, a place you enjoy, or an activity that was fun. Allow yourself to feel this good feeling of appreciation or care. If you can't feel anything, it's okay; just try to find a sincere attitude of appreciation or care. Once you've found a positive feeling or attitude, you can sustain it by continuing your Heart Focus, Heart Breathing, and Heart Feeling. It's that simple.

Although any positive emotion can elicit heart coherence, mature, intelligent love usually works the fastest. Love takes courage, which is at the heart of bravery and integrity. At a warrior resilience conference, a strapping Marine regimental sergeant major, unfamiliar with heart coherence, was connected to computer feedback that monitored his heart rhythms. At first, in front of the large audience, his heart was in the red zone (heart incoherence). He was asked to close his eyes, breathe calmly, and then re-create a time when he felt appreciation, value, purpose, or joy. His normally low pulse rate got even lower, and his heart rhythms quickly went to green (heart coherence). After this dramatic demonstration, I asked him what he had thought about. He said he was thinking of visiting his wounded warriors and their families. He said, "My heart and soul is there."

Practice the basic heart coherence skill several times a day. Try it when you awaken and when you go to bed. At first, try it when you are calm to gain confidence. Use it before, during, or after a stressful situation—when you want to perform well, recharge, calm down, think clearly, or comfort yourself. The skill tends to synchronize the heart with the brain and gut. A coherent heart also tends to positively affect the brains of others who are nearby, because of the heart's powerful electromagnetic field. So try this as a family or as a team before performing a difficult task. If you have the means you might also purchase technology that lets you monitor your heart rhythms on your computer or a handheld device in order to assess your progress (see the resources at the end of this booklet).

Calm Thinking

The thoughts that we habitually choose affects our arousal levels more than we usually realize. It works like this:

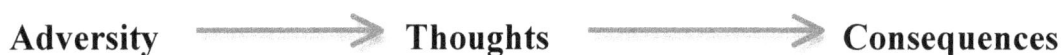

Adversity ➝ **Thoughts** ➝ **Consequences**

Most people think that adversity (a difficult situation) leads directly to negative consequences, such as arousal, impaired performance, or a bad mood. In fact, the thoughts that we habitually choose have a much greater influence. Say, for example, that teammates Bud and John botch a training exercise. Bud gives it some thought, determines how he will improve, and then lets it go. John stews about it, thinking, "What's wrong with me? I should have known better. I always get things wrong." His thoughts keep him aroused, so that he sleeps poorly and wakes up in a bad mood and distracted the next day.

Bud and John are equally capable. But along the way, John has picked up a habit of negative thinking. He has picked up thought traps called *distortions*—or unreasonably negative automatic thoughts. These thoughts pass through John's mind so quickly that he hardly notices them, let alone stops to challenge them. Because we are human and imperfect, we all think in distorted ways at times. These distortions can not only cause and maintain arousal, but also cause and maintain depression, anxiety, low self-esteem, and many other problems. Distortions are typically locked up in traumatic

16

memories, keeping these memories emotionally charged. The good news is that, through practice, people are capable of calmer, clearer thinking. We can learn to fairly quickly identify, challenge, and replace distortions—resulting in lower arousal, better mood, and better performance. More good news: there are only a handful of distortions that are linked to arousal and all the stress-related problems we've discussed. Learn these distortions well, so that under pressure you can readily catch yourself using them—and replace them with calmer, more functional thoughts.

The Distortions[iii]

Here are the distortions, along with calmer replacement thoughts.

1. **Flaw fixation.** Zooming right in on what is wrong, or what went wrong, and ignoring the positive aspects ("All I can think about is my screw up"; "Look at what you did wrong!"). Instead, try thinking, "I won't allow a negative element to overshadow all the good fortune around me." Ask, "Is it really the negative element that is ruining things for me, or my choice to dwell on it?" Ask, "What could I focus on to enjoy; what would I see if I were having a better day; what *isn't* wrong?"

2. **Dismissing the Positive.** Negating the positives, which might otherwise lift mood and self-esteem. ("Oh, anyone could have done that—it's no big deal," rather than, "I did a good job under the circumstances.") Instead of "Yes, but I could have done better," say "Thanks," and think, "Yes, I really do deserve some credit for juggling so many demands, getting all these difficult tasks done, working hard, getting most things done well, etc." See which approach motivates more.

3. **Assuming** (or jumping to conclusions without testing the evidence). There are two types:
   - **Mind Reading** ("I know he's angry at me.") Instead, ask! Check it out. Think, "Maybe it isn't so; I won't know until I ask. Maybe there's another possibility."
   - **Fortune Telling** ("I know I won't enjoy the party"; "I know I'll do poorly") Expect the middle ground, rather than extremes. Think, "I won't know for sure until I experiment. I'll probably have some success/enjoyment, as opposed to none. I might even surprise myself."

4. **Labeling.** Giving yourself (or another) a name or label, as though a single word could describe a complex person completely—*always* and in *every* case ("I *am* a dud"; "He *is* a loser"). Instead, rate behavior, not the person ("He is *driving* poorly"). Remind yourself that no one is always anything (dumb, rude, inept, etc.), and the person probably is already suffering from his/her faults. Ask yourself why someone's faults should bother you or why you should punish the person further. Apply the same standard to yourself.

5. **Overgeneralizing.** Concluding that your negative experience applies to all situations ("I *always* flop"; "I *never* succeed"; "*Everybody* hates me—*nobody* loves me"; "Nowhere is safe"; "Nothing means anything"). Instead ask, "What is the evidence that I never do well and always do poorly?" Or, "What's the evidence that all people fit this profile?" Instead, use words like "sometimes, often, generally, usually, yet" (e.g., "I haven't mastered this *yet*"). Test the notion that you never do well; experiment and see how well you do (your *performance* is likely to be somewhere between 0 and 100).

6. **All-or-None Thinking**. Evaluating yourself in extremes—allowing for no middle ground ("I'm a hero or a loser"; "I'm on top or a flop"). Instead, rate *performance or behavior*, not people (e.g., "I batted .750 today—my *performance* wasn't so hot"). A baby has worth, even though he/she doesn't perform well. Ask yourself, "Why *must* I bat 1000?" Accept the fact that those who don't win gold medals are not worthless, just human. (In fact, athletes who aim for an excellent job have been

---

[iii] Drs. Aaron Beck and Albert Ellis originally described these distortions. Some would argue that certain distortions are helpful in the war zone, such as "Distrust everyone you don't know." Upon reflection, however, it is clear that distortions don't usually help and don't transfer well to life outside the war zone.

found to perform better than those who shoot for perfection.) Remember that all people have both strengths and weakness at the same time, and still have worth. Enjoy the satisfaction of knowing you did your best, even though the outcome falls short of perfection.

7. **Unfavorable Comparisons**. Magnifying another's strengths and your weaknesses, while minimizing your strengths and another's weaknesses ("Bill is brilliant. I'm just average. Sure, he has a drinking problem and lots of people like me, but he's the one that *really* gets things done."). To counter this distortion, don't compare. Allow that each person is different and contributes in unique ways according to unique strengths (e.g., the contribution of a front-line soldier, a nurse, or a homemaker is no less valuable than a commander, doctor, or CEO, just different).

8. **Catastrophizing**. Making things much worse than they really are. ("This is awful and horrible. It couldn't be worse. I can't stand this!") Things really *could* be much worse and I *can bear* this, even if I don't like the inconvenience. If I don't avoid facing the difficulty of this challenge, I'll probably figure out a way to deal with it. Also, ask, "What are the odds of this 'awful' thing happening?"; "If it does happen, how likely is it to do me in?"; "How well am I preparing for or coping with this situation? (I'm probably somewhere in the middle, not at 0 coping.)"

9. **Emotional Logic**. My feelings "prove" that's the way it is ("I feel bad/inadequate/too tired to move. Therefore, I must be inadequate, incapable, unlovable, a loser, etc."). Remember that emotions are signals of upset, not statements of fact. Acknowledge the feelings, and allow that feelings change. Think, "Isn't it interesting that I'm experiencing this strong emotion. Don't go ballistic. It might change with rest, exercise, time, etc." If you feel worthless or bad, try to put a number to the reality (e.g., asking "What would 100% worthless or bad be?" helps avoid all-or-none thinking).

10. **Should Statements**. Rigid, unchallenged demands of ourselves and the world (e.g., "He *should* know better"; "He *must* not behave that way": "I *ought* not to tire, mess up, get depressed, be afraid, etc."). At least some of the problem is my expecting the world to agree with my perfectionistic expectations. People really are just the way they *should* be, given their beliefs, distortions, experience, breeding, etc., and it's foolish to demand they be otherwise. It *would* be nice if they were different, and maybe I *could* influence them to change. In fact, maybe I would motivate myself more effectively if I used more "woulds", "coulds", and "want to's" (e.g., "I *would like to* improve, and *want* to, rather than I *should*").

11. **Personalizing**. Seeing yourself as more responsible or involved than you really are ("It's all my fault that my son is failing in school"; "That guy is trying to aggravate me"). Distinguish influences from causes. Look realistically for influences outside of self (e.g., Instead of "What's wrong with me?" think, "The test was hard, I didn't prepare adequately, I was tired from working overtime, etc." In other words, focus on behavior and externals without judging self. Also, depersonalize ("Maybe I'm not the central figure in the other person's drama today").

12. **Blaming**. Putting all responsibility on externals, making us feel helpless ("This job is ruining my life and turning me cynical"; "I'm the way I am because of my crummy childhood"). Acknowledge outside influences, but take responsibility for your own welfare. ("OK, I understand how these things have influenced me. Now I commit to get back on track and move on." Or, "Nothing makes me do anything—I choose how I respond.")

Identify and Replace Drill

The first column in the pages following lists distortions that might go through a warrior's mind. As an exercise, cover up the second and third columns and see if you can first identify and then replace the distortion. The third column only lists options. There might be others. Working alone or with a buddy, see if you can discover more options that will be useful under pressure.

Thought	Distortion	Calm Replacement Thoughts
You stew about a mistake, forgetting about years of dedicated, mostly successful service.	Flaw Fixation	What didn't I do wrong? Maybe when my life is over people won't judge me solely by this isolated instance.
Nobody except my combat buddies can relate to what I've been through.	Overgeneralizing	Some people might. Some might try, and perhaps understand imperfectly.
God won't forgive me for what I did over there.	Mind reading	Where is that written?
I should have been able to save my buddy.	Should statement	Shoulds gives the illusion of control that I didn't have. I only have the power to do my personal best.
Either all my troops come home safely or I'm a failure.	All-or-none	I'll feel satisfaction in knowing I'll do everything that I can to protect them, and recognize that I can't control everything. Sometimes the enemy is very good at what they do.
I know my spouse is upset with me. She thinks I'm stupid.	Mind reading	I'll calmly check it out by asking. She could be upset at a lot of other things.
Your dissing me is personal.	Personalizing	Maybe this is more about his pain and less about me. I don't need to prove myself to him.
The enemy is worthless, incapable, and bad through and through.	Label	He has a different point of view. Respecting his abilities will prevent my becoming overconfident.
I trust no one. In the war even women and children carried grenades.	Overgeneralizing	Some people are trustworthy, some are not, and some are in between. I'll be alert to the differences.
I'm not as capable or brave as Joe.	Unfavorable comparison	Why compare? I have different strengths. It would be better to concentrate on doing *my* best, rather than *the* best.
I can't bear to think about my buddy's death.	Catastrophizing	Then I'll never grieve my loss. I'll do my mission, and then deal with my feelings later, when it's appropriate.
I feel so bad about what happened. I must have done something wrong.	Emotional logic	I feel sad about what happened, but I did my best.
I must always be hypervigilant.	Should statement	I can be flexible, and relax at proper times in order to recharge and be sharper.
That war screwed up my life.	Blaming	That was a difficult time. I'm going to make the best of that experience.
My anger feels justified. It must be.	Emotional logic	Maybe I'm not justified in taking my anger out on everyone, or excusing my bad behavior.
I should have been better.	Should statement	What do we really know when we are ____? (Fill in the age when you were imperfect.)
My buddies think I'm a loser for freezing.	Mind Reading	Maybe they think I'm human. Maybe they realize the difficulty to making a perfect decision in chaos.

I shouldn't be stressed about this.	Should statement	It would be good to be calmer. With more experience perhaps I will be.
I feel so anxious, I must be going crazy.	Emotional logic	Even those who reach their "breaking point" usually recover with time and rest.
I lost three men in that battle.	Personalizing	I didn't lose them. They were killed by the enemy.
I must not show fear.	Should statement	Survival isn't about not feeling fear—it's about acknowledging it and then turning it into productive, determined behavior. Some fear might enhance my judgment and performance. Even if I freeze, I'll breathe, and focus on what I intend to do.

Practicing

Remember that distortions pass through our minds automatically and habitually. We have to slow things down in order to catch and replace the distortions. When you feel disturbed by an event, try this exercise. Fill out a sheet of paper that looks like this.

Adversity_____

Consequences_____

Thoughts	Distortions	Calmer Replacement Thoughts

First, describe the event (adversity). Then describe the consequences (physical and emotional). In the first column, list separately the upsetting thoughts that went through your mind, or go through your mind now as you think about the event. When this is done, label each distortion that you identify in the middle column. In the third column, write a calmer replacement thought for each distortion. Then see if the intensity of the emotional consequences decrease somewhat.

You can do this at the end of the day, or any other time when things settle down. It can be very effective to try this in pairs, with a buddy asking questions, such as: "What happened?"; "How did that "make you" feel?"; "What thoughts went through your mind?"; "And what else went through your mind?"; "Are any of these thoughts possibly distortions?"; "Could this thought possibly be a ____distortion?" The buddy can then help brainstorm replacement thoughts. In this buddy exercise, both get better at replacing distortions with calmer thoughts.

Underlying the distortions are what are called core beliefs. These are deeply held beliefs that are learned at a very young age. Core beliefs come in two basic types: *I'm inadequate* (incapable, powerless, out of control) or *I'm unlovable* (not good enough, flawed, bad). As an exercise, try to consider reasons or evidence as to why these core beliefs are unreasonable. For example, "Sometimes I have been quite capable, such as when I _____"; "Everyone has some likeable traits (such as willingness to try, persistence, caring, etc.)."

Four

Managing Distressing Emotions

During the course of our work and our lives, adversity will inevitably trigger strong negative emotions, such as fear, grief, anger, sadness, or guilt. Although they are to be expected, such emotions can overwhelm your resilience if you don't have skills to effectively manage them.

Emotions are part of what make us human. They are helpful, not bad. For example, fear can alert us to danger and trigger the right amount of stress to improve performance. Within limits, anger can energize us and help us to persist in a good cause. Grief is an expression of love that helps us to come to grips with losses so that we can carry on better. If we shut down our ability to feel and learn from negative emotions, we will also shut down our ability to feel positive emotions like happiness and love.

Of course, problems arise when strong feelings build and we don't know what to do with them. Like a pressure cooker, they might build and build until they explode in destructive ways. We might try to avoid or run from negative emotions with alcohol, painkillers, adrenaline rushes, risky behaviors, or excessive work, gambling, thoughtless sex, TV, computer games, or buying. Of course, none of these do anything to change the root emotions. Inner pain might erupt in domestic violence, fighting, or other ways that leave the original pain untouched, The goal of this chapter is to help you be more aware of your emotions, and then to manage them in the right way at the right time. The pattern is to be aware of your emotions, understand what they are telling you, suppress strong negative emotions when you need to accomplish a mission or task, and then process these emotions when the time is right until they subside. For example, you might notice yourself becoming aroused and use this awareness to remind yourself to do tactical breathing. Later, when things settle down, you might use the skills in this section to give the strong emotions that you suppressed the attention they need.

Note that the skills in this chapter will ask you to initially work with moderately distressing memories, so as not to be overwhelming. As you gain confidence in a skill, you might eventually try it with a more distressing memory. If in doubt, or you feel you need assistance, discuss your concerns with a mental health professional.

Defusing[iv]

The psychologist Steven Hayes notes that almost everyone suffers intense pain sometime, such as depression, anxiety, self-dislike, even battling thoughts of suicide, at some point in life. One sharp Marine told me that he wished he could take a laser and erase his painful memories of Vietnam. However, erasing our histories from memory isn't possible, and the more we try to fight or flee the memories, the more emotionally charged they become. What is needed is a change in tactics! In defusing, we fully join the battle, letting pain into full awareness, only this time with a completely accepting and kind attitude. Then we step away from the battle and move on with our lives, without wasting energy trying to change the memory.

1. *Identify a moderately painful memory.* Perhaps you'll recall a situation that made you feel embarrassed, rejected, shamed, disrespected, angry, hurt, abused, ridiculed, inadequate, or unloved. Perhaps you made a mistake or a bad decision. Perhaps you were mistreated. Maybe a

---

[iv] This section is adapted mainly from Hayes, S. C., with S. Smith. (2005). *Get Out of Your Mind and Into Your Life: The New Acceptance and Commitment Therapy.* Oakland, CA: New Harbinger Publications. Also, Hayes, S. C., K. D. Strosahl, with K. G. Wilson. (1999). *ACT: An Experiential Approach to Behavior Change.* New York: Guilford Press.

parent or "friend" labeled you lazy or a coward, and you've tried to run from that memory for years. Maybe you experienced adversity more recently.

2. *Write down how that situation bothered you.* Describe the thoughts, feelings, images, and bodily sensations.

3. *Write down how long the memory has bothered you?* Has thinking gotten rid of it?

4. *Pick a single word that describes what the memory makes you feel about yourself.* The word might be: *bad, inept, dumb, loser, helpless, powerless, inadequate, coward, lazy, disgusting, shame, guilt, stupid, clumsy*, etc.

5. *Rate how distressing that word is, from 1-10.*

6. *Now, welcome that memory into full, accepting, kind awareness*—not as an enemy you are fighting, but as a friend you are welcoming into your home. Not with the thought, "I'll grit my teeth and tolerate this for a minute so I can get rid of it," but rather, "I welcome this memory fully into kind awareness." Let your body be soft and relaxed.

7. *With this kind and open attitude, repeat aloud the single word that you selected in step one as many times as you can for 45 seconds.* When finished, re-rate the distress level. Notice what has happened. Do you notice that the word loses some of its emotional impact—it's just a word? Do you feel less fused with the word? Is the memory and/or the word less distressing? Do you realize that you really *can* bear it? If so, this might be a good skill to use with other distressing experiences. It is powerful to invite our pain into open, kind awareness, and notice how the way we experience the memory shifts.

You can try this again, this time varying how you repeat the word. You might say it loud, then soft. Slow, then fast. Falsetto, then low in pitch. Try it in a scolding tone, like nasty old Aunt Edna would use, then in a playful tone. These variations can further help to change the way you experience the memory.

Rapid Relief Techniques[v]

The next two techniques can be very useful to gain temporary and fairly rapid relief from intense, distressing emotions. Such emotions might arise from adversities ranging from an argument with the boss or a spouse to getting shot at or witnessing a traumatic scene. For overwhelming or potentially overwhelming emotions, it is best to try these techniques within the context of a therapeutic relationship with a trauma specialist. For events involving moderately intense emotions, you might experiment with these on your own.

Eye Movements

This technique, described by Dr. Larry D. Smyth,[vi] is not to be confused with Eye Movement Desensitization and Reprocessing (EMDR), a comprehensive treatment for PTSD and other stress-related mental disorders. Eye movements help about two-thirds of people who try it. The instructions follow:

---

[v] This and the following sections are adapted from Schiraldi, G. R. (2009), *The Post-Traumatic Stress Disorder Sourcebook*, New York, McGraw-Hill, 2009.

[vi] Eye movements was developed by Dr. Larry D. Smyth, Sheppard and Enoch Pratt Hospital, as a useful adaptation of Dr. Francine Shapiro's eye movement desensitization and reprocessing. Detailed instructions are found in L. D. Smyth, *Treating Anxiety Disorders with a Cognitive-Behavioral Exposure Based Approach and the Eye-Movement Technique: Video and Viewer's Guide*, Havre de Grace, MD: RTR Publishing, 1996. ©1996 by Larry Smyth, Ph.D.

1. *Identify a past or present situation that distresses you and is difficult to shake*. Remember, go easy. Do not try this at first for a situation or memory that is extremely intense for you. Rather, pick a moderately distressing event at first to gain confidence in the technique. While this technique does not usually lead to negative side effects, there is always the possibility that one might be overwhelmed by trying to go too fast too soon. In a moment you will think about the situation to the point that you feel five to six subjective units of distress (SUDs), where 0 means you feel pleasantly relaxed with no distress, and 10 is the most intense discomfort you could possibly feel.

2. *Imagine the upsetting situation*. Notice the feelings, bodily sensations, images, and thoughts that go along with this. Stew about it, adding the negative thoughts ("Oh no....this is the worst...why did this have to happen?") until the SUDs level reaches 5-6. Don't' allow the SUDs to go higher, because we don't want this to become overwhelming. A level of 5-6 is moderately distressing—uncomfortable but tolerable. At this level you can think clearly.

3. *With eyes open and head still, move two extended fingers of a hand back and forth*. The hand is about 14 inches in front of the eyes, and the back and forth movement covers a distance of about two feet. Move back and forth about twenty-five times.

4. *Notice where your SUDs are now*. Typically you might notice them drop to 4-4 ½. Notice any shifts in the thoughts, images, bodily sensations, and/or emotions. People often notice that thoughts, emotions, or bodily sensations change or lessen in intensity, images shrink or fade, etc. If your SUDs dropped a little, then this technique seems like a useful skill for you. Repeat the back and forth movements.

5. *If you wish to use this in places where back and forth hand movements are inconvenient, be creative*. You might pick two spots on the wall or on your knees and move your eyes between those spots. You might wish to move your eyes back and forth with your eyes closed, or with your hand over your eyes as if you were in deep thought.

6. *If this technique dropped your SUDs, try practicing it several times a day over a one*-week period to gain mastery of the skill. Use it as a rapid stress reducer when you want to soothe your nerves, or perhaps before returning home from work.

Thought Field Therapy

Thought Field Therapy (TFT) is another simple technique that can bring rapid relief from strong and distressing emotions. Its originator, Dr. Roger Callahan (a WWII vet), asserts that it is a self-help technique that can decrease emotional distress related to anxiety (including panic, phobias, worries, fears), depression, stress, troubling memories, guilt, grief (e.g., from death or a broken relationship), fatigue, and embarrassment. He notes that it also dramatically improves heart rate variability (which is related to heart coherence) typically within minutes, while helping to reduce pain and symptoms of certain chronic diseases, such as fibromyalgia and asthma. There are, he states, no apparent risks or side effects—it either works or it doesn't. One using the technique does not have to talk about, analyze, or disclose any details regarding the adversity. The technique is easily learned and can be taught easily to others. Thus, you can become a greater resource for others. Preliminary research in Kosovo, Rwanda, and elsewhere appears to support the favorable clinical impressions regarding its use. The instructions that follow are an adaptation developed by Dr. Robert L. Bray.[vii] In this technique, you will tap solidly with the balls of two fingers of either hand—firmly but not so hard as to be

---

[vii] Adapted with permission from modifications of Robert L. Bray, Ph.D., LCSW, Director, Thought Field Therapy Center of San Diego, www.rlbray.com .

uncomfortable. To prepare, locate the tapping points as follows (it does not matter which side of the body you use):

1. *Side of hand.* This is fleshy part where one would do a karate chop.
2. *Under nose.* Between the lip and the nose.
3. *Beginning of eyebrow.* Just above the bridge of the nose.
4. *Under eye.* On the bone about an inch beneath the pupil, when looking straight ahead.
5. *Under arm.* On the side of the torso, about four inches below the pit of the arm.
6. *Under collarbone.* Place your two fingers at the notch at the base of your neck. Drop your fingers down an inch and slide them over about an inch.
7. *Little finger.* Along the nail line on the inside of the finger, next to the ring finger.
8. *Under collarbone.* Same as in step 6.
9. *Index finger.* On the nail line on the side near the thumb.
10. *Under collarbone.* Same as in step 6.

The *gamut spot* is so-called because you carry out a sequence of activities while continuously tapping there. Make a fist, then place the index finger of the tapping hand between the knuckles of the little and ring fingers. Slide the index finger an inch toward the wrist. You'll tap this gamut spot, while the hand being tapped is flat.

Here are the instructions for TFT:

1. *Think about/remember a situation that had a moderately negative impact on you.* Rate the upset, using SUDs ranging from 1-10. If you can't remember a situation, focus on an image, feeling, sensation, or sound.
2. *Tap in succession each of the ten major points about 6-10 times:*
    a. Side of hand
    b. Under nose
    c. Beginning of eyebrow
    d. Under eye
    e. Under arm
    f. Under collarbone
    g. Little finger
    h. Under collarbone
    i. Index finger
    j. Under collarbone
3. *While continuously tapping the gamut spot, do the following:*
    a. Close eyes
    b. Open eyes
    c. Look down and left
    d. Look down and right
    e. Whirl eyes in circle
    f. Whirl eyes in circle in the opposite direction
    g. Hum any tune
    h. Count to five
    i. Hum again
4. *Repeat Step 2 above.*
5. *Re-rate upset. Repeat the whole sequence (steps 2-5) until there is no further drop in the upset.* Stop if there is no drop in upset after several repeats.

6. *End with floor to ceiling eye roll if the SUDs rating is two or less.* That is, while tapping the gamut spot and holding your head level, rotate your eyes on a vertical line from floor to ceiling over a period of 6-7 seconds.

Why Do These Techniques Work?

There are various theories as to why these techniques can be effective. First, both techniques help us to confront the pain. Exposing ourselves to distress is the first step toward desensitizing the nervous system, whereas avoidance maintains memories and resulting arousal. Stimulating both sides of the brain helps the brain process distressing memories that are "stuck." It is likely that the brain already contains thoughts and images that help to neutralize distressing memories. More fully activating the brain likely stimulates the healing process. Both techniques disrupt racing, worrisome thoughts—and focusing on bodily sensations, either by noticing them or by tapping, tends to ground one in the body and calm. Further, in tapping energy meridians, TFT is thought to unblock energy "perturbations."

Writing What's Wrong

Research has shown that old emotional wounds, even in soldiers, don't necessarily heal with time. Unresolved, they can exert an influence that affects present health and functioning for many people, regardless of when the traumas were experienced.

The psychologist James W. Pennebaker reasoned that "keeping it all inside" is not healthy. Undisclosed wounds that are not processed and expressed verbally often intrude painfully into awareness and find expression in bodily and psychological symptoms. They also compete with attentional resources, degrading mental functioning.

Pennebaker asked various groups, ranging from students to survivors of the Holocaust, the San Francisco earthquake, the Gulf War, and job firings, to simply write about their most difficult adversities. He instructed them to put down their deepest thoughts and feelings surrounding the event, writing continuously for 15-30 minutes on each of four days. Pennebaker was surprised by the amount of traumas experienced by people who appeared "normal" on the outside. Traumas ranged from accidentally causing deaths to rape, physical and sexual abuse, and being blamed for parents' divorces. Childhood traumas were least likely to have been confided, and the most likely to cause illness later in life. Those who confided in writing showed better physical and psychological health afterward. Understandably, mood slipped during the four days of writing. Thereafter, those who disclosed showed less depression, anxiety, and stress, while experiencing greater self-esteem, stronger immunity, and fewer illnesses. Those who had lost their jobs found new employment quicker if they had written about the firing. Writing about past adversities has also been linked to improved sleep, job satisfaction, working memory capacity, and grades, and reductions in symptoms of arthritis and asthma.

Slowing down to put our painful memories into words helps the brain organize, neutralize, complete, and settle them, so that they can be stored like normal memories. People who write about their troubling memories often report that they understand them better and are less troubled by them, being more able to move on. People realize that they can express their feelings, even with tears, and then return to a stronger normal. The process can be likened to opening a bullet wound in order to help it drain and heal.

Confiding in writing seems to particularly help those who have never told anyone about a distressing event (e.g., for fear of embarrassment or punishment), but wish they had or could have. You might try confiding in writing for any past trauma or adversity that still troubles you, including the loss of a loved one, a break-up, moving, parents divorce, or anything else you'd like to forget, avoid, or resolve. It is comforting to realize that we can confront what we have run from, and in so doing overcome our aversion to the memories.

Dr. Pennebaker offers the following guidelines for disclosing in writing[viii]:

1. *Getting ready to write.* Find a time and place where you won't be disturbed. Ideally, pick a time at the end of your workday or before you go to bed. Promise yourself that you will write for a minimum of 15 minutes a day [15-30 minutes usually works well] for at least 3 or 4 consecutive days. Once you begin writing, write continuously. Don't worry about spelling or grammar. If you run out of things to write about, just repeat what you have already written. You can write longhand or you can type on a computer. If you are unable to write, you can also talk into an audio recorder. You can write about the same thing on all 3-4 days of writing or you can write about something different each day. It is entirely up to you.

2. *What to write about.* Something that you feel is affecting your life in an unhealthy way. Something that you have been avoiding for days, weeks, or years. Something that you are dreaming about. Something that you are thinking or worrying about too much.

3. *Instructions generally given in Dr. Pennebaker's research:*

    Over the next four days, I want you to write about your deepest <u>emotions and thoughts</u> about the most upsetting experience in your life. [Start by describing the facts, then the emotions and thoughts.] Really let go and explore your feelings and thoughts about it. In your writing, you might tie this experience to your childhood, your relationship with your parents, people you have loved or love now, or even your career. How is this experience related to who you would like to become, who you have been in the past, or who you are now?

    Many people have not had a single traumatic experience but all of us have had major conflicts or stressors in our lives and you can write about them as well. You can write about the same issue every day or a series of different issues. Whatever you choose to write about, however, it is critical that you really let go and explore your very deepest emotions and thoughts.

    Warning: Many people report that after writing, they sometimes feel somewhat sad or depressed. Like seeing a sad movie, this typically goes away in a couple of hours. If you find that you are getting extremely upset about a writing topic, simply stop writing or change topics.

4. *What to do with your writing samples.* The writing is for you and for you only. Their purpose is for you to be completely honest with yourself. When writing, secretly plan to throw away your writing when you are finished. Whether you keep it or save it is really up to you. Some people keep their samples and edit them. That is, they gradually change their writing from day to day. Others simply keep them and return to them over and over again to see how they have changed.

5. *Here are some other options:* Burn them. Erase them. Shred them. Flush them. Tear them into little pieces and toss them into the ocean or let the wind take them away.

Some Other Tips

• Use a rich range of emotions, both negative and positive as you write. Naming emotions calms the amygdala. Use statements such as "I feel sad because…"; "I feel like my world shattered"; "I was so scared that…" Younger men especially might have to persist longer in order to feel comfortable with this technique. Rather than using slang, try to name genuine feelings (e.g., sad, disappointed, hurt, humiliated, lonely, angry, caring, eager, excited).

[viii] Adapted with permission from Dr. James Pennebaker's website:
http://homepage.psy.utexas.edu/homepage/Faculty/Pennebaker/Home2000/WritingandHealth.html

- Try to add insight words (e.g., *realize, know, understand*) and causal words (e.g., *reason, because*). The use of such words in writing is tied to greater benefits.
- It is good to use writing for adversities that you can't control, especially if you can accept having imperfect control.
- If you feel distressed after writing, remember to try the techniques you have learned so far: abdominal breathing, progressive muscle relaxation, heart coherence, eye movements, or thought field therapy.
- Remember, if writing is overly distressing ease up. Approach the event gradually or write about a different topic.
- On the fourth or fifth day, you might also discuss in writing how you have or could have benefited from the adversity. What good can come out of this experience? What lessons, if applied, would make this event more meaningful? What advice would you give to an imaginary friend undergoing a similar situation regarding how to deal with this adversity? Were there bright spots in the darkness? (Did you somehow persevere and show certain strengths? Did you or others demonstrate nobility of character?) Could you give the story a new twist—could the event signal a new beginning with a positive ending?
- If writing about a traumatic event doesn't help, see a mental health professional who specializes in treating trauma. A trauma specialist will help you learn other healing strategies. As with the other techniques in this book, you might also seek the help of a mental health professional if you feel that remembering the event might be too overwhelming.
- Writing about present day concerns (worries) has also been found to be very useful. If simply trying to "relax and stop worrying" isn't working, try writing about what is worrying you (facts) and what you are feeling and thinking. During the day, postpone worrying until your next "worry period", when you can write about your worries for about 25 minutes.

The bottom line is this*:* If you want to reduce distress, try keeping a journal that no one but you will see. Write the facts, thoughts, and feelings regarding either past adversities or present worries. It is rare to find that such a simple, inexpensive strategy can be so effective. Remember to add this tool to your coping strategies.

Managing Distressing Dreams

Many warriors who experience a traumatic event, even those who don't develop PTSD, are troubled by recurring nightmares. Nightmares disrupt sleep, raise arousal levels, and often cause fatigue and impaired performance the next day. Of course, for those with PTSD, nightmares increase suffering. So dream management is an important skill for service members. Think of a nightmare as simply distressing memory material that needs to be processed and settled, not avoided. The principle is to bring all aspects of the nightmare into calm awareness and to change both our response to the nightmare and the nightmare itself. Here are the steps:

1. *Normalize them.* Nightmares are a very common result of being exposed to very distressing events, such as combat, witnessing death or injury, abuse of any kind, rape, or a perceived personal failure that leads to guilt or shame. Nightmares are the brain's attempt to sort out and make sense of the event. Common themes occur in nightmares. It can be reassuring to just realize that many others have experienced these themes. Dr. Deidre Barrett, a Harvard psychologist and president of the Association for the Study of Dreams, and her colleagues have identified the following themes and symbols in nightmares:

- Danger
- Monsters
- Being chased
- Being rescued
- Dying
- Revenge
- Being threatened again by an assailant or other traumatic event
- Being punished or isolated
- Being trapped or powerless
- Sexual abuse (dreams might include shadowy figures, snakes going in holes, worms, blood, good and bad sex, injury, being trapped, being paralyzed, shame, guilt, anger, violence or death)
- Filth, excrement, and garbage (can symbolize evil, lack of purpose or dignity, disgust or shame)
- Physical injury (losing teeth is fairly common, which might symbolize losing control, being powerless or unattractive, or being wounded emotionally)
- Being visited by the deceased

2. *Realize that nightmares require attention.* Normally, dreaming helps to process and settle challenges that we are facing. However, when one is depressed or for highly disturbing memories, processing can get stuck as the nightmares recur. (Recall that cortisol impairs the brain's ability to store memories properly.) Avoiding the memory material doesn't work. Neither can our normal active, problem solving coping methods change what happened. Instead, we can turn toward the nightmare and process it until the memory loses its emotional intensity.

3. *Confide your dreams.* Sometimes all that is needed to diminish the intensity of nightmares is to share your dreams verbally with a supportive person or in a journal. Verbalizing in a supportive environment helps to neutralize the intense emotions and integrate the memory fragments—so that the entire memory can be settled. Notice that the confiding process is similar to that described in the previous section, Writing What's Wrong.
   - Relax and describe your dream in detail. Break it down into the following specifics:
      - What is the setting?
      - Who are the characters?
      - What is happening?
      - What are you doing? Feeling? Thinking? What are your physical sensations?
      - What are the symbols?
      - What are the symbols saying?
   - Create a system to recall your dreams. You might not remember the content of your dreams, especially if you are not in the habit of paying attention to your dreams. You might keep a dream journal to help remember the details of your dreams. You might keep a pad of paper and a pen, or an audio recorder, beside your bed.

4. *Rehearse a different, calmer response.* Imagine that you see yourself at a specific, intense point in the dream carrying out a simple task, such as looking at your hands, and saying in the dream, "This is just a dream." Practice this before you go to sleep, to serve as a cue to remind yourself that this is just a dream, should the dream recur.

5. *Modify the nightmare in an appropriate way.* Starting with dreams of lesser intensity, you might, for example:
   - Confront the monster chasing you and ask in a direct and friendly way, "What is it you want—what are you trying to tell me?" One person confronted the monster and discovered

that it represented himself and his guilt. He assessed his guilt and made some growth-promoting changes. See if you can make the monster laugh or smile, or get it to dance.

- Create a new ending. For example, see yourself performing better, or your unit rapidly rescued. A combat veteran sees his buddy, "now with God, standing guard and smiling." You might simply visualize yourself saying, "I am safe now, I survived," or any other positive thought. Write out or talk out what you did. Rehearse the revised dream in your imagination for about 15 minutes daily for a week.

- Using art to draw the nightmare can be very effective. Some find it is easier to talk about memory material once it is on paper, "out there" at a distance. Once you have drawn pictures relating to your dreams, try to discuss them or write about them in a journal, since verbalizing helps to settle the memory material. You need not be good at art: even children can do this very effectively. Simply:
  - Draw the nightmare—what is happening.
  - Draw your body and how it is feeling physically and emotionally. You might write down the thoughts that go through your mind as you look at the picture.
  - Draw the more positive ending.
  - Draw your new physical and emotional reactions (and what you think when you look at this new ending).
  - Draw your new choices. You might draw a safe place, or you relaxing or traveling in calm safety, or you moving ahead in a good way with your life.

6. *Expect changes in dream content.* As we bring memory material into the light of day, we allow the brain's natural healing process to "reboot", or start again. You might realize you did the best you could under those difficult circumstances. Dreams of the deceased might include assurances that they are now well off or opportunities to say good-bye. You might now dream of more positive outcomes. Dreams might begin to shift in focus to everyday concerns. You might simply feel better, sleep better, or feel brighter about the future.

Five

Especially for Warriors

Deployments to war zones present special challenges, especially when repeated or extended. Resilient warriors are as well prepared emotionally as they are physically for war and its aftermath. This chapter will help you anticipate and prepare emotionally for deployment. If you have returned from deployment, this chapter will help you make more sense of your experience.

Confront Worst Case Scenarios: Emotional Inoculation

In medicine, injecting (or inoculating) people with small doses of germs allows them to build immunity. Likewise, exposure to smaller doses of emotional stress allows service members to gradually build emotional strength.

You might study books that realistically describe the experiences of warriors, such as *Lone Survivor* (Marcus Luttrell), *Two Wars* (Nate Self), *With the Old Breed* (E. B. Sledge), and *From Vietnam to Hell: Interviews with Victims of Post-Traumatic Stress Disorder* (Shirley Dicks). Some excellent movies are *Saving Private Ryan, We Were Soldiers,* and *Blackhawk Down.* If you have returned from deployment, these resources will likely help you view your experiences in a different light—perhaps helping you to understand and normalize them.

Another very effective approach is to think of the most stressful event that you could possibly face. Perhaps you have already experienced such an event, or can imagine it. For example, you might think of watching a buddy die or accidentally causing the death of an innocent civilian. With a buddy, discuss the events you identified and then pick one to work on. In writing, describe: (1) the facts about the event; (2) how you would likely respond to the event (what you would think, feel, and do before, during, and after); (3) how most service members would respond to this event (describe thoughts, feelings, and behaviors before, during, and after); (4) what you would consider an ideal response (discuss thoughts, feelings, and behaviors before, during, and after); and (5) how you would feel if your response were less than ideal. When both of you are finished writing, exchange your written responses. Each person reads the other's responses. Then discuss what you observed or have learned from the other person's writings. This exercise can literally be life saving as buddies explore a range of coping options, some of which they'd never before considered. You might see that even strong warriors can be uncertain about their coping ability, but that all can improve their emotional coping confidence with practice. You'll likely build a greater sense of teamwork as you work together to improve your coping abilities.

On Killing
> *...every time I kill someone I feel farther away from home.*
> Tom Hanks' character in *Saving Private Ryan*

For many, killing is the most stressful aspect of war. Failing to acknowledge this prevents us from preparing for killing's emotional aftermath. Army Ranger and former West Point psychology professor Lt. Colonel Dave Grossman explains that those who train to kill must reconcile with the reality of killing, or *suffer more afterwards.* With permission, we'll summarize Grossman's main points on killing.[ix]

[ix] Adapted with permission from: Grossman, D. (1996). *On Killing: The Psychological Cost of Learning to Kill in War and Society.* New York: Back Bay, © 1996 David A. Grossman; Grossman, D., with Christensen, L. W. (2004). *On Combat.* Millstadt, IL: PPCT Research Publications, ©2004 David A. Grossman; Grossman, D. (2009, February 26). *Bulletproof Mind.* Training presented at International Critical Incident Stress

1. *Killing is traumatic*. In all wars since WWI, there have been more psychiatric casualties than deaths from enemy fire.
2. *Most Americans find killing repugnant*, and would rather befriend and build than harm others. Even enemy combatants are viewed as fellow warriors and humans. It is normal to feel revulsion and guilt after killing. Yet killing can destroy you emotionally if you haven't thought it through.
3. *Many warriors raised in the Judeo-Christian culture have been taught, "Thou shalt not kill"* (Ex. 20:13). However, in nearly all Bible translations, the original Hebrew word *ratzach* is more correctly translated as "murder." Murder is the unlawful taking of life with malicious intent (e.g., for personal gain). Thus, it is not killing that is prohibited, but murder. In fact, the Bible frequently mentions war, killing, and soldiering without condemnation—and honorable warriors, such as Joshua, Gideon, and the Roman centurion found God's favor. Honorable warriors commit and prepare to fight violence to protect those who can't defend themselves and society's most cherished values. They are commissioned by their government to lawfully use lethal force when required for these purposes.
4. *Warriors who are prepared to legitimately use deadly force decisively and without hesitation—with the assurance that their cause is just—can better live with having killed afterwards.* If you've worked through in advance the moral, spiritual, and emotional aspects of killing, you'll be less likely to be traumatized afterwards. Elite warriors, such as U.S. Navy SEALS, generally suffer less psychologically after war, in part because they have reconciled with killing. Note the SEALS creed, which states:

   > In times of war or uncertainty…a special breed of warrior [stands] ready to answer our Nation's call…to serve his country, the American people, and protect their way of life…always ready to defend those who are unable to defend themselves…I voluntarily accept the inherent hazards of my profession, placing the welfare and security of others before my own…We train for war and fight to win. I stand ready to bring the full spectrum of combat power to bear in order to achieve my mission and the goals established by my country. The execution of my duties will be swift and violent when required yet guided by the very principles that I serve to defend.

Preparing to kill for a just cause takes sober reflection, good judgment, and experience. It begins with stopping avoidance and fully facing the issues involved. Grossman's stages of killing is a very useful place to start:

1. *Self-questioning*. The combatant asks, "Am I capable of killing? What if I freeze and let my buddies down?" Killing is often more frightening than the fear of being killed. Being a coward and letting one's buddies down is another of combatants' biggest fears.
2. *The actual killing*. The warrior does what he is trained to do, often automatically and under the influence of a surge of adrenaline.
3. *Exhilaration*. The warrior has hit the target, executed his combat duties, and saved lives. He often feels euphoric, exhilarated, and relieved, knowing that he performed well and has survived. He might be in the state of denial—saying that he is fine, while manifesting a 1000-yard stare.
4. *Aftereffects*. The magnitude of killing hits. One might feel like a destroyer who has committed the ultimate sin of taking life. Perhaps the act seems even worse as the combatant approaches the fallen enemy and finds pictures of family, or hears the dying enemy cry, "Mom!" At this stage, remorse is common. Perhaps the combatant feels guilty for feeling satisfaction. Here he must distinguish between satisfaction from doing his duty (which is healthy) and satisfaction from killing (which is not). I once interviewed a hunter whose family needed the meat that he provided. He felt satisfaction in providing food for his family, but always felt queasy about

---

Foundation 10th World Congress on Stress, Trauma & Coping, Baltimore, MD. The section "On Being Wounded" also reflect his thoughts.

taking the deer's life, even though he felt it justified. A similar, but more intense, conflict is typical among warriors who kill. The surviving warrior might typically ask, "Where do I stand before God?" and might feel that innocence and joy have been lost. Nausea, sleep disturbance, flashbacks, depression, anxiety, and dissociation (we'll cover this shortly) are commonly experienced. After killing, warriors might feel as if they are hovering above the scene of the killing or feel that the scene is happening to someone else. It is not uncommon to have distorted memories about the killing. Some feel bad for freezing, even though this is sometimes prudent to prevent unnecessary killing, or understandable when the warrior is taken by surprise and is uncertain of what to do. Some shake to realize they could have been killed.

Negative aftereffects are minimized if the warrior has worked through killing beforehand, remembering that satisfaction comes from preserving life and freedom, not killing. Other useful ideas:

- I'd chose not to kill, but the enemy makes the decision as to whether or not I use deadly force.
- I'll do what the government trains me, equips me, authorizes and empowers me, and expects me to do.
- God won't reject me for lawfully killing when necessary." (Alvin York, the most decorated soldier in WWI, was a conscientious objector for religious reasons at the start of the war. After an officer explained to him, from a Biblical perspective, the need to use lawful killing to stop tyranny, he became a committed, noble warrior.)
- A warrior deters evil and ultimately saves lives.
- I'm prepared to confront people who hurt others.
- The enemy intends to kill my friends and me, and will do so if I don't take decisive action.
- I think I'm going to have to kill this guy. He thinks he can take on the might of my government.

5. *Rationalizing and Acceptance.* If one hasn't worked out killing beforehand, this might be a long process. As Grossman says, "Combat kills enough people. It's madness to let it destroy me mentally, too." Honorable warriors have sworn to fight evil. They are motivated by profound love. Warriors who kill usually do so in the context of trying to protect others. This stage is completed when the warrior realizes that sometimes the enemy needs to be killed for the good of society; force was justified and necessary. If you feel guilty that a comrade fell in battle, remember that warriors accept that unavoidable risk—the fallen comrade would want you to go on and live joyfully. It is helpful if elders remind the warrior who has killed, "You did your duty for a good reason. Welcome to the club." The enemy wins if survivor guilt takes out another honorable warrior.

A hallmark of PTSD is avoidance. The opposite of avoidance is acceptance—fully facing reality. Warriors learn to come to terms with the necessity of lawful killing. They learn to approach war with determination and confidence, not avoidance. The following training considerations can help:

1. *Make targets as human as possible.* This helps combatants adjust to the idea of pulling the trigger on another human being when required to do so. Training with rapid response software can help you reduce unnecessary shootings, while applying lethal force more effectively when required.

2. *Mentally rehearse killing the enemy.* In today's violent world, the enemy might be children who have been programmed to hate, or terrorists dressed as civilians. Visualize the scenario before, during, and after killing. Include details such as remembering the morality of the fight, picking a point to aim at, seeing the mortally wounded enemy, walking off the adrenaline afterwards, and remembering helpful thoughts. As uncomfortable as this may seem, it is better to mentally rehearse than to be caught unprepared and overwhelmed.

3. *Expect to handle killing better with training and experience.* Seasoned veterans are so called because years of experience help them maintain grace under pressure and bounce back emotionally. It is normal to find killing repulsive, especially at first. Eventually, the warrior accepts killing as a necessary action that duty requires. With determination, experience, and training, an area that is feared and avoided becomes an area of confidence.
4. *The honorable warrior accepts the world in a balanced way.* He accepts that there is evil in the world. Without honorable warriors, evil would prevail. He knows that if he is prepared to do his duty, he will do so with little panic. He will function better—being less likely to be killed himself and more likely to support his buddies who depend on him.

Reflections on Killing
- I asked a World War II veteran why he fought. He said, "I was 18 years old. I knew the difference between right and wrong. I didn't want to live in a world where wrong prevailed…so I fought." (Steven E. Ambrose, author of *Band of Brothers*, remarks at the dedication of the National D-Day Museum, June 6, 2000)
- The only thing necessary for the triumph of evil is for good men to do nothing. (Edmund Burke (1729-1797), British statesman and philosopher)
- Except for ending slavery, genocide, Fascism, Nazism, and Communism, war has never solved anything. (Anonymous)
- If there must be trouble, let it be in my day, that my child may have peace. (Thomas Paine (1737-1809))
- If you must kill, do so out of a sense of duty and justice, never with hatred. Hatred carries a heavy price. (Anonymous)

On Being Wounded

If you are wounded, keep going without panic. There are many recorded cases of warriors fighting back and recovering after being hit by multiple bullets. If you know you are wounded and alive, it shows you can still think and function. Stay calm and focused on what you want to do. Resolve that you will live and stay focused on why you want to survive. Forty percent of one's blood can be lost without losing consciousness. You might experience racing heart, dry mouth, and sweaty palms, yet you can still likely carry on. If afterwards you experience anxiety, nightmares, flashbacks, or other stress symptoms, this is normal. Remember the skills you've learned to reduce stress, such as calm breathing, thought field therapy, eye movements, and journal writing.

War Zone Integrity

Abuse no one and nothing, for abuse turns the wise ones to fools and robs the spirit of its vision.
Tecumseh, Shawnee Warrior

No man, deep down in the privacy of his own heart, has any considerable respect for himself.
Mark Twain (who struggled with depression)

How we choose to behave in the war zone will largely determine whether we return with regrets or inner peace. Committing and witnessing atrocities has been found to predict PTSD, suicide, and guilt in combat vets upon returning home. Atrocities—cruel, brutal, or evil behaviors— include:
- Unlawful violence: killing, torturing, or humiliating civilians or enemy prisoners.
- Stealing from civilians or the enemy.
- Rape, which cheapens the perpetrator's sexuality and makes it more difficult to experience wholesome intimacy. Rape also typically traumatizes the victim for decades (PTSD, sexual

disgust, fear of intimacy, and a range of physical symptoms including pelvic pain, gastro-intestinal disorders, and headaches are common).

- Following unlawful orders.

Atrocities, whether committed by Nazis or prison guards at Abu Ghraib, embolden the enemy. In addition, they haunt and corrupt the spirit of the perpetrator. Moral wounds are typically accompanied by shame, self-loathing, and loss of inner peace. Some returning vets incite brawls, demanding from others the respect they don't feel for themselves. Or they seek to cover their pain through work, sex, drugs, or other highs. Numbness might alternate with anger, depression, and anxiety. Conversely, right actions strengthen one spiritually, resulting in self-respect, spiritual wholeness, and confidence.

Paths to Inner Peace and Self-respect

The wise warrior will think through the moral aspects of the war zone in advance in order to prevent long-term scarring of the soul. There are two pathways to inner peace and self-respect:

1. *Decide in advance to live morally—then do so.* Determine what you will and won't do. Previously developed codes might aid this process. For example, in their creed, SEALs pledge to "Serve with honor on the battlefield…Uncompromising integrity is my standard. My character and honor are steadfast. My word is my bond…The execution of my duties will be…guided by the very principles that I serve to defend." Let your actions be guided by justice and duty, never hatred or vengeance. This will minimize regrets. Beware of gradual entrapment, or seduction by degrees, regarding your conduct. For example, the seemingly harmless belittling of the enemy might eventually lead to treating them inhumanely. Respect the enemy's humanity and intelligence, if not his cause.

The Warrior's Code of Honor

- I will always act in ways that bring honor to my comrades, my cause, and me.
- I will use lethal force when duty requires without hesitation—and only when duty requires.
- As much as humanly possible, I will show concern for innocent human life and the welfare of enemy combatants who are no longer a threat.
- I will speak the truth, knowing that lies in battle cost lives.
- I will distinguish between right and wrong, choosing the harder good over the easier wrong.
- I will be motivated by loyalty to my comrades, duty, and the justice of my cause, and not revenge.

---

2. *When you err, have a system in place for righting wrongs.* Humans will always be imperfect, and will always make mistakes. The Army's *Combat and Operational Stress Control Manual for Leaders and Soldiers* states that even well trained individuals in highly cohesive units might make bad decisions under extreme combat and operational stress. Try to live beyond reproach. If you slip, remember that no one is beyond redemption. Most world religions have a method for making peace with wrong actions: Admit the wrong, make amends when possible, acknowledge mitigating circumstances, reconcile with Deity (e.g., allowing God to take away the burden), resolve not to repeat the misconduct, and forgive yourself for being imperfect (releasing the desire to punish yourself and be burdened by regrets).

Reflections on War Zone Integrity
- Great individuals make great teammates. (John Wooden)
- Every atrocity strengthens the enemy and potentially disables the service member who commits it. (Jonathan Shay)

- Do the right thing when you are out there. (Vietnam vet struggling with PTSD, imploring his buddies)
- The steady trigger finger kills a lot more enemy than the one that trembles with hatred (Lt. Colonel Dave Grossman)
- A peace above all earthly dignities, a still and quiet conscience. (Shakespeare)
- What stronger breastplate than a heart untainted! (Shakespeare)
- A person of good character feels moral pain after doing something that caused another person suffering…even if entirely accidental or unavoidable. (Jonathan Shay)
- Somewhere, at this very moment, there is a Soldier in training…who is preparing for war and expects a leader of character…The American Army is a force for good—each of you will be a force for good. (Lt. Gen. William B. Caldwell, IV)
- We should neglect no honorable means of dividing and weakening our enemies. (Robert E. Lee)
- No one has the right to do wrong, not even if wrong has been done to them. (Viktor Frankl)

Dr. Edward Tick, a psychotherapist who has treated many war veterans, asserts that PTSD is best understood as an identity disorder and soul wound—with moral pain being a root cause. The following essay is based on his book, *War and the Soul: Healing Our Nation's Veterans from Post-Traumatic Stress Disorder.*[x] It captures many of the themes and challenges of trying to be an honorable warrior. Please read the essay, and then complete the activity at the end.

On Being an Honorable Warrior

The soul (*psyche* in ancient Greek) is deeper than the intellect. The soul reasons and rises above instincts. It yearns and searches for meaning, ethics, beauty, love, harmony, and order. The soul dreams; it chooses between good and evil. War, however, can trigger our uncivilized nature—unkind and brutal instincts which may as yet be unrestrained. It can shatter our sense of goodness and innocence, and leave one feeling like someone different, separated from the soul.

Universal Warrior Themes
In nearly every generation and culture there are recurring themes centered around war, warriors, and conflict—and their potential for good and bad. For example, the Greek pantheon had two war gods: Athena used war rationally and reluctantly in order to protect civilization, resulting in spiritual triumph. She did not delight in war's horrors. Ares, on the other hand, the god of slaughter, was bloodthirsty, undignified, and unrestrained.

Saint Augustine reasoned that war should only be used for good intentions, "securing peace, punishing evil-doers, and uplifting the good" and never motivated by "the passion for inflicting harm, the cruel thirst for vengeance, an unpacific and relentless spirit,…or the lust of power."

The Ideal Warrior
Most cultures depict honorable warriors as being on a spiritual journey, embodying the finest virtues of humankind, despite war's violence. Honorable warriors are servants of civilization, defending and protecting causes they consider dearer than self or personal gain.

Preparing for war is a rite of passage that can, as William James wrote, propel one constructively into adulthood by building toughness, maturity, discipline, tolerance for discomfort, and higher functioning. Among Native Americans, capable warriors earned respect and recognition, while those who didn't pass the test honorably felt alienated and unproven as men.

---

[x] Adapted with permission from Tick, E. (2005). *War and the Soul: Healing Our Nation's Veterans from Post-Traumatic Stress Disorder.* Wheaton, IL: Quest. © 2005 Edward Tick.

Having faced death, honorable warriors understand how fragile life and happiness are, and thus strive to preserve peace. They will try to avoid conflict unless their homeland and cherished values can be protected in no other way. They will not profane life or dishonor the dead, but will treat others with dignity and respect.

Honorable warriors direct their abilities actively, persistently, and bravely, with mind and body in harmony. They rise above the warrior's shadow traits—avoiding malice, cruelty, impulsivity, emotional unsteadiness, rage, and sadism, which can be unleashed in war. Thus, they do not kill with hatred or vengeance, but only as duty requires. Dr. Tick notes that the North Vietnamese veterans have much lower rates of PTSD than American soldiers suffered. Significantly, Ho Chi Minh told his people not to hate or blame American soldiers, but to only consider them as victims of their leaders' decisions.

War Wounds and the Warrior's Soul

In order to go to battle with the whole heart, the warrior must believe the threat to be a real threat to his homeland, loved ones, and/or most cherished values—one that can only be resolved through armed conflict. False pretenses lead to moral wounding.

However, even in a war considered just, the warrior's soul can still be damaged. "No man in battle is really sane," said William Manchester, a WWII Marine vet in the Pacific. War requires one to be violent, perhaps to kill another person who in another time or place could have become a friend. Veterans commonly ask, "Am I good or bad? Did I murder? Will God forgive me?"

Even in wars whose cause is considered suspect, warriors might feel respect for enemy soldiers slain in a fair fight and experience no guilt. However, random killing of innocent civilians or the committing of atrocities (e.g., torturing prisoners of war, raping, stealing, or maliciously destroying property) leads to regrets and deeper, lingering moral pain.

Also, witnessing the carnage of war can cause one to become numb or indifferent to the suffering of others, which is contrary to the ideals of the honorable warrior.

Rejecting the Warrior Identity

The reality of war's horrors can lead warriors to deny, disown, shun, or squash their warrior identity. The warrior might feel different since returning from the war, or separate from his or her soul. The soul might feel diminished, shattered, lifeless, or wounded. But rejecting this part of the soul also disconnects us from the power for good of the warrior's soul.

Reclaiming the Honorable Warrior

Veterans are not necessarily warriors just because they have been to war. To become an honorable warrior, one learns to bring forward war skills into present life in a mature way.

In peacetime, the honorable warrior uses acquired wisdom and vision to build and protect life, rather than to destroy it—dissuading people from the use of violence, unless it is absolutely necessary. Honorable warriors fearlessly keep sanity and kindness alive in their homeland.

As they did before the war, they stand for life, justice, and beauty. They cultivate character, kindness, compassion, honesty, decency, cooperation, and sensitivity to the suffering of individuals.

They accept and affirm conflict and war's hardships. Their souls become big enough and loving enough to contain these.

On the battlefield, they show restraint and resist dehumanization. That is, they do not mix the violence of war with hatred, cruelty, and impulsivity. They treat prisoners and the wounded humanely. After the war, they hold no grudges, but are forgiving so that they can live in the present. In contrast, dishonorable warriors are insecure, still trying to prove themselves. They remain hardened to the suffering of others and thus prone to cruelty. They are unable to control their aggression, and are hostile and impatient with imperfect or weak people.

After war, honorable warriors apply their skills in the service of humanity, perhaps becoming police, firefighters, or politicians. They see themselves as belonging to the human race, and not a tribe.

Thus, they might return to war-torn countries to rebuild schools or hospitals, or to provide medical supplies or assistance. They view former enemies as brothers and sisters who now share a common experience.

The mature warrior distinguishes murder (which is unauthorized, vengeful, hateful, or malicious homicide) from killing in battle. For example, in the Judeo-Christian tradition, waging war for power or personal gain is considered wrong, but fighting to preserve the survival of loved ones is not.

Conclusion

Moral wounds can worsen the wounds of PTSD and keep them festering. From the standpoint of prevention, therefore, it is wise for each potential combatant to:

- Be clear on why you are fighting and reconcile to the necessity of the conflict and violence.
- Determine in advance to only do what you consider to be good behavior, and to refrain from doing bad in order to minimize regrets that can plague your conscience.
- After the war, use your warrior skills for the betterment of humankind.

Activity

As you consider the virtues of the honorable warrior as described above, please list five behaviors you will do during war, and five behaviors you will not do. Then list five ways that you will use your warrior skills and wisdom after returning from war in the service of humanity.

Being Ready for Stress Symptoms

Your training and life experience have taught you much. You will likely remain remarkably resilient most of the time. Be confident in your coping ability. But you are human, not invincible. Your resistance can be worn down over time. Combat stress symptoms are not a sign of weakness, but a signal to take care of yourself. Have a plan for taking care of symptoms. Know that the "heroes", those who never seem to show weakness, are sometimes the most vulnerable to combat stress because they don't know what to do when stress levels rise. Don't be surprised to find that certain events can stir strong feelings, such as seeing grotesque scenes (e.g., carnage or mutilated bodies, including children), the death of buddies, or being wounded. Should you find troubling symptoms starting to build:

1. *Remember to use your basic skills*: sufficient sleep, exercise, good nutrition, calm breathing, progressive muscle relaxation, heart coherence, calm thinking, thought field therapy, eye movements, defusing, journal writing, and dream management. Talk things over with a supportive person. Resist the common myth that no one cares or will understand. Avoid avoidance—escaping pain through drugs or alcohol, withdrawing, or addictions (excessive work, gambling, shopping, or risky behaviors).
2. *Distinguish guilt from shame.* Guilt is feeling bad about a specific behavior—either acting wrongly or failing to act rightly. Shame is feeling bad as a person, worthless to the core. Acknowledging realistic guilt is healthy and can lead to constructive changes. Shame is not healthy. Because you are human, you will make mistakes. Learn from them, but don't judge or condemn yourself for being imperfect. No one, no matter how imperfect, is worthless or beyond redemption. The goal is to accept responsibility for *realistic* guilt, do something constructive, and then release the guilt. Warriors often shoulder guilt for a long time for feeling glad they survived, performing below their training level (due to fatigue, confusion, uncertainty, fear, etc.), falsely believing that they can prevent all injury or loss of life, or being unable to control their stress symptoms. What they often fail to consider is how the brain, as remarkable as it is, is prone to miss or misinterpret information, lose focus, and make mistakes under great stress. If you feel burdened with guilt, try this exercise, suggested by VA counselor Raymond Scurfield:

Identify an event that triggered the guilt. Then make a list of all the people who share responsibility for the event. You'll likely list yourself, but consider all who played a role in this event, such as the enemy, leaders, politicians, buddies, those who might have inadequately trained or equipped you, etc. Next to each person, list the percentage of responsibility that he/she bears for the outcome. Then take a look at what you've written. If the total exceeds 100%, which is impossible, then adjust your ratings. Often, you'll end up decreasing the percentage of responsibility that you bear to a more realistic level. What do you do with the remaining guilt? Confront it in a kind, forgiving way. Sometimes warriors discuss difficult past events with buddies at reunions and learn that there were mitigating circumstances they'd been unaware of, or they gain a new perspective. You might come to accept how truly difficult it is to make cool and correct split-second decisions during the chaos of battle. You might forgive your imperfections and inexperience ("What did we know when we were twenty-two?"). You might dedicate yourself to helping others. Then forgive yourself and start anew, knowing that no one is worthless or incapable of growth. In chaos, mistakes happen. No one sees the whole picture, and no one is in a position to judge you. Mistakes do not define who you are or who you will become.

3. *Be prepared for dissociation.* Dissociation is quite common during or after battle. If unchecked, it can lead to PTSD and other problems. To understand dissociation, look at the figure below.

AWARNESS AND MEMORY (From Schiraldi, G.R., *The Post-Traumatic Stress Disorder Sourcebook*, New York, McGraw-Hill, 2009).

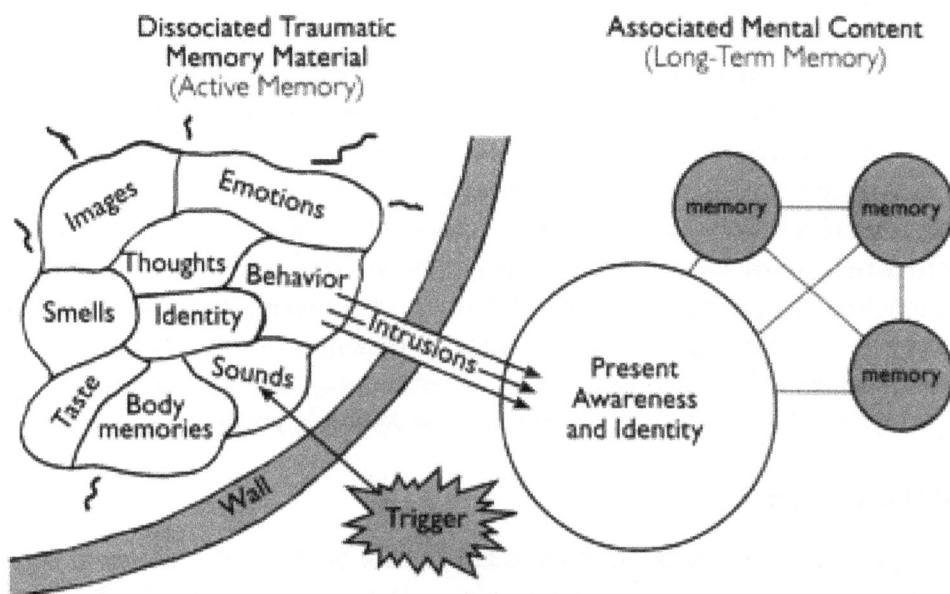

Normally the brain files memories in long-term memory, like files in a filing cabinet. The three circles on the right represent *associated* memories. You can pull such a memory into your awareness with appropriate emotion, know that it has a beginning and an end, and know when it occurred relative to other memories. Whenever you pull up an associated memory, you feel like you are the same person. And then you can file the memory away again fairly easily. A *dissociated* traumatic memory is stored differently—like it is always on the desktop. The dissociated memory is walled off from associated memories. It doesn't seem to have a beginning and an end. It remains highly emotionally charged, and the memory fragments don't hold together well, so that a reminder of the event (or trigger) pulls memory fragments into your awareness when you don't want it to. Thus, the smell of diesel while driving in a convoy might trigger the memory of an ambush and cause you to feel excessively aroused. Typically, distorted thoughts are part of the dissociated memory. These thoughts are usually unspoken and unchallenged, so they tend to keep the emotional charge of the memory high. Finally, your awareness or identity might "split." Either part of your awareness and identity might get pulled into the memory (as when something triggers a flashback), some of your awareness might drift away as you try to mentally "escape" from a painful memory or stressful situation, or you feel like two different people before and after the traumatic event.

You can recognize dissociation in yourself or others by the following:

- Depersonalization—mentally leaving the body and looking down on self or another victim to avoid suffering (e.g., "I was on the ceiling watching my wounded body.")
- Spacing out or drifting away (missing a conversation, being unresponsive to others, losing track of what's happening, withdrawing, falling asleep)
- Derealization—"I'm not here"; "It feels as though I'm in a dream"; foggy feeling; distorted sights/sounds; things move in slow or fast motion; feeling out of touch with surroundings; familiar places seem strange; not recognizing yourself in the mirror
- Flashbacks (suddenly and vividly experiencing the traumatic memory, or parts of the memory, as if it were recurring in the present)
- Numbness to pain or feelings
- Body becomes still or stiff
- Twitching, grimacing
- Attempts to self-soothe and stay grounded—rocking, jiggling leg, stroking chair
- Eyes stare downward or blankly (1000-yard stare), dart anxiously, or blink/flutter rapidly
- Disorientation
- Feeling split, like a different person since the trauma ("My husband's soul is still over there.")
- Sudden strong, unexplainable emotions or physical sensations
- Intrusive memories—especially when trying to relax or sleep, when stressed, or when drinking or using drugs
- Forgetting all or parts of the trauma, or portions of your life
- Experiencing different personality states, one or more of which may be attempting to contain distressing trauma material (this is uncommon and is usually associated with severe childhood trauma, such as sexual abuse)

Since dissociation can degrade performance and mental health, prevention and treatment of dissociation are critical. The following strategies help to manage dissociation:

1. *Treat unresolved past trauma.* Those who enter crisis situations with unresolved trauma are more likely to dissociate and develop PTSD. The goal of treatment is to fully process the dissociated memory material—merging the memory fragments and neutralizing the strong emotions and distortions, so that the memory can be stored alongside the other memories in long-term storage. Now the traumatic memory is experienced as just one memory on file, and not the one memory that constantly dominates awareness.
2. *Desensitize the nervous system.* Excessive stress arousal is linked to dissociation. Do the calming strategies we've already discussed. Especially remember calm breathing (hyperventilation can induce dissociation). Also try yoga, tai chi, and meditation, which we will discuss soon.
3. *Optimize brain health.* All the steps that improve brain health probably reduce vulnerability to dissociation: exercise, diet (remember especially to increase intake of omega-3s, fruits, and vegetables, and to reduce saturated fats and sugar), adequate sleep (sleep helps to process traumatic memories and probably reduces dissociative symptoms), avoid harmful

medications and drugs (including smoking, stimulants, and heavy or binge drinking), and regulate blood pressure.

4. *Manage panic.* Overwhelming fear can lead to panic attacks, which can lead to dissociation, which can lead to PTSD. Calm panic as follows:

- Pre-plan and practice self-instruction statements for *before* a crisis (e.g., "This could be rough, but I'll focus on my job."), *during* a crisis (e.g., "Fear is normal. Relax, take deep breaths and focus on what I need to do."), and *after* a crisis (e.g., "All in all, I did pretty well"; "It's OK to feel distressed. I'll mindfully walk it off and accept the emotions without judging them.").

- Calm your body. Relax your muscles and use calm breathing. Adapt a special approach to panic: Rather than tensing, which worsens panic, say, "Hello, fear." Bend with the panic attack like a reed blowing in the wind until the panic attack runs its course (usually within ten minutes). Focus on the job at hand and staying alive and functional. Calmly flow with, rather than trying to escape or stop, the fear. In other words, let the fear in, if it comes, with a soft, accepting heart. Avoid smoking, which greatly increases the risk of panic attack.

- Should dissociation occur, accept it without judging or fighting it.
  - Think, "Dissociation is just the mind trying to protect me from pain. Nevertheless, I'll bring awareness back to the task at hand."
  - Ground yourself. You can ground in your body by mindfully noticing clenched muscles and reminding yourself that this is normal. Relax with low and slow breathing. Rub something (such as fabric, your elbow, a tool, or weapon), wiggle your toes, or press your feet down—movement helps to expend stress. Also try mindfully walking off adrenaline or doing progressive muscle relaxation. You can also ground yourself in the surroundings. To prevent your mind from drifting away, describe five objects that you see around you in detail. Then describe five sounds you hear. Then physically handle five objects.
  - Talk to your buddies. Putting words to the experience helps to integrate traumatic memories.
  - If additional help is needed try eye movements or thought field therapy.

5. *After the crisis is over, allow time to decompress and calm down if possible to restore psychological order.* If traumatic memories intrude or you experience other symptoms of dissociation, ground in the present by telling yourself:

- "This is a memory from the past talking—old stuff. It will pass."
- "My feelings are understandable. They come and go."
- "I'm safe now."
- "That was then. This is now. Today is____. The time is _____."
- "I'm here now."
- "This is the same me—before, during, and after the trauma."

- *Ground in your posture.* In the book *Trauma Practice*, Dr. Anna Baranowsky and colleagues suggest this: Notice when you dissociate that you slouch, your face shifts, and you feel emotions such as fear, sadness, anger, and vulnerability. Exaggerate that posture, facial expression, and emotions. Now stand in a strong, confident posture and facial expression. Alternate back and forth between the negative and confident perceptions. Notice that you are in control.

- *Journal the facts and feelings to defuse and integrate the traumatic memories.* Some find that debriefing (discussing the various aspects of the crisis in a peer group setting) helps reduce the impairment resulting from dissociation.

- Use psychological first aid. In *Waking the Tiger*, Peter Levine explains that animals in the predator's jaw will freeze (or dissociate), as though dead. Should the predator drop its prey and go away, the animal will kick, twitch, and shake to restore equilibrium—and then run to safety. In a similar way, allow yourself to shake and tremble after the crisis. This is the body's way to release stress and counter the freeze state of unspeakable terror. One or two days after the crisis, try recounting the trauma. Ground in your body if the emotions become too intense. Allow yourself to tremble and shake, as this is normal. Try to complete and discharge the movement that was frozen during the trauma. Perhaps you see yourself moving differently and performing better. Thus, if you froze in an uncertain lethal force encounter, this time see yourself squeezing the trigger as you were trained to do. You might actually make the desired movements.

Know Thyself Activity

Make a list of the post-crisis stress symptoms you have encountered or would likely encounter. List the actions you will take to manage those symptoms.

Early Treatment Readiness

The resilient warrior is a master at rebounding. If you suffer from PTSD or any other stress-related disorders, remember that current treatments are very helpful at getting people back on track. Although getting needed help at any time can be effective, waiting might make recovery more difficult and increase the likelihood of developing medical illnesses. A number of generals and other high-ranking officers have recently acknowledged their struggles with PTSD and/or other stress-related problems—reporting that the professional help they got made them better leaders. "Suck it up and press on" works in battle. Afterwards, stop and admit needs so that you can heal and carry on better. Be flexible. Rigid trees break in the wind. You might liken a mental health professional who teaches new coping skills to a coach who teaches athletic skills. You'll likely come out of treatment with additional coping skills and more emotional confidence.

Acknowledging strong feelings, even fear, grief, and pain, shows that you are human, not weak. You unburden so that you can heal, move on, and return to full living. Some people fear that they'll lose control if they let their feelings out. Generally, you release strong feelings, and soon get back to normal. Losing control is more likely if you *don't* get needed help (e.g., erupting in anger, damaging relationships or a career). Denied pain calls out for healing and often doesn't go away with time. Find needed help if what you are doing to get back to normal isn't working. Some mental health professionals don't understand combat stress. But some do. Look until you find someone who is right for you (see the resources at the end of the book). Your eligibility for a security clearance will not be affected if you receive counseling for issues strictly related to marriage and family problems (excluding violence), grief, or adjustments from service in a military combat environment.

Six

Homecoming

Coming home at last! A time of happiness. A time of adjustments.

You'll likely return home changed. You'll probably feel different than you were and different from those who have not deployed. It will take time to get used to life at home again, and you and your loved ones will adjust better if you know what to expect.

In short, readjusting to life at home will take patience and flexibility. Things may not return exactly to the normal you remember. However, they can return to a satisfying "new normal" that respects all the ways that you and your loved ones have changed. Allow yourself time to adjust. It might take a year or longer to get back to normal, or to reach a new normal.

You'll probably realize that your family has changed in your absence. They've been holding it together without you, fearing for your safety—and that's been hard. They've probably established new routines, and become more independent in doing so. Self-reliance is good, but it might make it hard for them to adjust to your expectations when you return. Young children might not warm up to you quickly. Stress might interfere with sexual intimacy. This, too, might require time in order to restore comfort, warmth, and trust.

Take time to reconnect to people you left behind. Take time to get to know new friends, whose freedoms you have defended. While everyone may not appreciate what you have done, many will. You have a right to rejoin the country and community you sacrificed for.

Warriors in all times have struggled to meet the challenge of homecoming. You only have to read Homer's *The Iliad and the Odyssey* to realize that the challenges for warriors haven't changed much throughout history. Both you and those you associate with need to understand that homecoming is a process. Both you and the civilians you served need to be patient with each other and the transitioning process. As you are patient and understanding, others will more likely reciprocate.

The warrior needs two sets of skills: war zone skills and home life skills. War zone skills are powerful survival skills and ways of thinking. Because of the life and death intensity of war, these skills become deeply etched in the warrior's mind. These skills don't often transfer to life at home. War isn't normal. The skills that are normal in the war zone are not often normal at home. It can be very useful to understand these war zone skills (please see table below).[xi] Next to each skill area is a war zone skill(s). The third column shows how a war zone skill can cause problems at home. The fourth column suggests goals for homecoming, when situations are usually less critical.

Skill Area	War Zone Skill	Can Translate at Home to:	Goals for Homecoming
Safety	Stay constantly alert/vigilant (e.g., don't let your guard down, even in "safe zones," because of infiltrators).	Fear of traffic jams; irritation when something is out of place; checking locks often; being uncomfortable in crowds; must sit with back to wall; can't relax when others do; overprotective of loved ones; don't understand casual attitudes.	Gradually turn down vigilance so that you are appropriately watchful, but can relax more when it is safe to do so.

[xi] Based on *Transitioning War Zone Skills* by Dr. James Munroe, Boston VA Healthcare System, james.munroe@va.gov.

Skill Area (continued)	War Zone Skill	Can Translate at Home to:	Goals for Homecoming
Distrust	Suspect everyone, except those who are well known and proven; be suspicious.	Being overly suspicious & distrustful; suspecting people's motives; not allowing others to provide needed help—all of which interfere with building close relationships.	Aim for the middle ground; begin to trust more readily unless given a reason to doubt one's motives; assume that people are innocent until proven guilty.
Anger	Apply swift, aggressive responses, which can save lives. Strong anger and foul-language are the war zone norm.	Angry and aggressive responses to traffic, assumed disrespect, or children playing on your property; you go from calm to rage quickly; you don't tolerate disagreements. Your anger frightens children, pushes people away, and leaves you isolated.	Turn down the frequency, intensity, and duration of anger, knowing that anger frightens those who are close to us. If people complain about trivial things (e.g., a hard bed, traffic) just think, "That's just people being normal."). Lighten up over others' imperfections. It's not usually critical.
Unpredict-ability	Be unpredictable because predictability kills (e.g., vary routes; don't tip your hand).	Not relaxing on holiday; refusing to be where you're expected to be; refusing to be on time.	Try to give loved ones the security of knowing they can count on you. Let them know your plans.
Intelligence	Don't let intentions be known, be cautious about what you say; be wary of social chatter.	Keeping to yourself even in close relationships. People must guess what you like or dislike, and what you are thinking or feeling. You may not tell loved ones where you're going or when you'll return.	Share more of what you feel and think as trust levels build. Learn to enjoy being yourself again.
Mission Orientation	One clear, life-and-death mission gets total focus and energy. Intolerance for lateness.	Everyday things seem unimportant, and may not get attention until they reach crisis levels. Once you lock on to a "mission", you may have difficulty releasing it until it's completed. You may get excessively irritated at lateness.	Find enjoyment and rhythm in everyday routines again. Chores that maintain the home are not trivial. Be patient with others. Work hard, but also relax and refresh. Remind yourself, "It's not life or death."

Skill Area (continued)	War Zone Skill	Can Translate at Home to:	Goals for Homecoming
Decision Making	Decisions are not overly discussed, and are carried out by those of lower rank without question or much discussion. Indecision costs lives.	You expect others to follow your orders without questioning, and get frustrated when people don't, or when they want to discuss/talk things over.	Realize that there is usually time to talk things over. Shared control generally makes both spouses happier. The goal is not always to make a decision or be in control, but to promote growth, respect, and closeness. Respect your family's independence—it helped them survive your absence, and will help them survive in the future. Strive for interdependence—freely chosen, not mandated.
Response Tactics	Respond automatically— act first, think later; don't hesitate. Everything must be in its place and ready to go. Then respond forcefully, and instill fear in the enemy.	Anger when something is not in its place, rooms are messy, or dishes are dirty. You may seem unfriendly or intimidating to others. Intolerance of incompetence.	At home it's usually best to think first, then act. Allow time to weigh choices, which avoids impulsive behaviors. Loved ones respond better when they feel secure, not afraid.
The Enemy	People are either with you or against you. When in doubt, assume they're enemies.	Everyone is seen as an enemy. This stance interferes with making new friends, building intimacy, and getting along with co-workers. It also keeps you isolated, and makes it difficult to mingle socially.	Realize that it takes time and effort to get a good read on people and build relationships. There is time to do this. Be willing to risk; let people in.
Emotions	Become numb or turn off feelings (fear, horror, disgust, or grief) so that you can function. Showing emotions is seen as a weakness in combat. If you get too close, you get burned when your buddy is killed—so put up a wall.	You don't read emotional signals of your family so you don't know how to respond. You don't relate/empathize. You don't feel positive emotions either, and don't have fun. You seem cold and uncaring, or bored. You turn to risky behaviors to feel something (e.g., adrenaline rush).	Showing emotions at the appropriate time is a sign of being human, and shows caring. Recognize emotions in others and feel with them in order to empathize and be close. It's good to learn to relate at the feeling level. Gradually allow yourself to be close and vulnerable more often. This is safe to do at home. Express love often in words.

Skill Area (continued)	War Zone Skill	Can Translate at Home to:	Goals for Homecoming
Authority	Distrust of incompetent or immoral leaders.	May resent or overly challenge those who have authority over you, such as a boss.	Accept that even incompetent leadership at home is probably not a life or death situation.
Loss	You become hardened to loss. There's no time to mourn losses—another mission calls.	You miss comrades who had your back in the war zone, but you don't grieve. You're seen as cold and unfeeling. You might even avoid normal loss rituals.	Accept grief and funerals as a normal part of life that helps people say goodbye and adjust to loss.
Talking	It's OK to boast about war stories, but not to talk about what it really was like for you inside.	You are likely more comfortable talking with, or drinking with, your buddies but not your family or helping professionals. This might make your loved ones feel excluded.	Gradually risk with people who are trustworthy and respectful. See if that doesn't build connections. Keep military friends, *and* widen your circle of social supporters.

Difficult Questions

When you come home you'll probably be asked questions about your experience, such as "What was it like. Did you kill anyone?" How you respond will depend on many factors, including who is asking, how they are asking (e.g., is it genuine concern, is it thoughtless chatter, or is it an invitation to criticize you?), when and where they ask you, and how prepared you feel to answer. A range of responses is possible. You might choose not to answer at all, give a partial answer, or give a more thoughtful answer. You might discuss this with people you trust, such as buddies, family, or helping professionals. You might prepare some responses such as:

- Vets don't usually talk about that.
- I don't know how to explain it.
- It was difficult. Most Americans would rather befriend, but it was my duty.
- Maybe sometime I'll tell you about it, but this isn't the right time.
- It was our duty. I wear this uniform. Whoever is better gets to go home.
- When my number was called, I did it.

If people disrespect you, don't be surprised. Dissent has been a part of every war. Be calmly and inwardly proud that you defended even their freedom of speech, stood between them and evil, and were willing to sacrifice even for them. You have nothing to prove to dissenters.

Re-deployment

Learn about the culture you will deploy to. Perhaps study their history and language. Warriors generally are more comfortable and respectful among people they understand.

Seven

Happiness

What does happiness have to do with warrior resilience? Plenty! Growing research has found that happiness is central to health and performance. Happiness correlates strongly with resilience, and in the opposite direction with anxiety, depression, anger, and other indicators of mental distress. Happy people thrive more *occupationally* (e.g., earning more; being more productive, energetic, and flexible; enjoying their career more), *socially* (having more friends, less divorces, and greater satisfaction with family), and *medically* (living longer, and suffering fewer colds and many other medical conditions). They adapt to and recover better from adversity, such as depression and grief. Positive feelings also stimulate brain growth and hasten recovery from arousal—while helping people to see a broader range of coping options. So happiness is an important survival skill for warriors, and a force multiplier.

What Is Happiness?

Happiness is what most people around the world say they want most. Happiness is two things: (1) Inwardly feeling positive emotions on a fairly regular basis (e.g. contentment, inner peace, calm, serenity, awe, hope, enthusiasm, love, and amusement), and (2) The overall feeling of satisfaction with one's life and oneself—that these are worthwhile and meaningful. So happiness is not a fleeting feeling, but a more consistent, inner condition and ability to enjoy life—even when things around us are chaotic. While it's impossible to always be happy, happy people spend less time feeling down, and know how to bounce back when they do feel down.

It turns out that on average nearly half of happiness is in the genes, and only 10% is related to all outer circumstances combined, like income, physical attractiveness, climate, age, gender, race, religious affiliation, marital status, education, or passive entertainment (e.g., TV). That means that 40% of happiness can be influenced by what we regularly think and do, and our attitudes.

Who Is Happy?

Certain cultural factors are associated with happiness. Once people's basic needs are met, money does not affect happiness much. In fact, many lose their happiness trying to obtain more and more. While married people are generally happier than unmarried people, it appears that happy people are more likely to get married and stay married. In other words, happiness before marriage might lead to more satisfying and enduring marriages. Those who marry with the steepest expectations of marriage (e.g., expecting perfection of their partner), while having the fewest marriage skills, experience the steepest declines in happiness. Being politically conservative and living in a democracy are consistently associated with greater happiness.

Aside from living in a democracy, being politically conservative, and working at a good marriage (which gives a small bump in happiness in several studies), what increases happiness? First, ask your doctor about ruling out or treating medical or psychological disorders that can affect mood, such as depression, PTSD, anxiety, sleep apnea, thyroid imbalances, and elevated cholesterol. Beyond this, there is much that can be done to increase happiness. Building happiness takes advantage of brain plasticity—the fact that we can build new neural pathways in the brain that are associated with greater happiness. Here are the pathways to happiness supported by the research.

Self-Esteem

Around the world, self-esteem is strongly correlated to both happiness and resilience. It is usually the strongest predictor of happiness. Wholesome self-esteem protects against depression, while those lacking in self-esteem are more likely to experience PTSD, anxiety, depression, shame, and arousal under stress.

How we define self-esteem is critical. Self-esteem is a *realistic, appreciative* opinion of oneself. *Realistic* means that we are honestly aware of our strengths and weaknesses. *Appreciative* means that we have an overall positive regard or feeling about self—a quiet gladness, despite being imperfect. Warriors who are secure in their worth don't need to boast or prove themselves to others. They remain humble, knowing their limits, but are generally confident about life.

Self-esteem is built on three foundation stones:

1. *Unconditional worth as a person.* Someone might have more *market* or *social* worth than you or I, but core human worth comes with birth. Social and market worth might result from externals, such as income, rank, appearance, marital status, acquired skills, the car one drives, or the unit one belongs to. Such worth can rise or fall according to our good or bad performance, the way we are treated, awards, promotions or demotions, or transfers. By contrast, worth as a person is unchanging and anchored in something deeper—who we are at the core. Each person, at birth, comes with a set of capacities—all the attributes and potentials needed to live well. Thus, each person has the capacity to reason, learn, sacrifice, love, enjoy, and contribute. Each of these qualities exists in embryo, capable of being grown. It is the unique mix of strengths that make one person different from another. Inner worth already exists; it doesn't need to be created or proved. It is not lost by imperfect performance, being mistreated by others, or having an illness. Each person is literally worthwhile, meaning they are worth the time it takes to live well and actualize their potential.

2. *Unconditional love.* Effective parents communicate to children that they are loved, no matter what, and this love provides the secure foundation for their growth. While these parents care enough to set limits, the child understands that mistakes won't lose their love. Note that love from others does not *make* one worthwhile, although it might help one to *feel* worthwhile. A great task in life is to learn to love unconditionally. If you didn't learn to do this from your parents, you can still learn to be unconditionally loving to yourself. Love is more motivating than self-condemnation and harsh criticism, and makes growing more enjoyable. There is no survival value in self-hatred whatsoever.

3. *Growing* is the process of actualizing our strengths—becoming more capable, caring, and productive, and elevating self and others. Although fruitful living doesn't create or increase inner worth, it definitely helps one to feel more satisfied with oneself and one's life course. We enjoy growing as an expression of who we are, not to prove our worth. Growing is the process of doing one's personal best and feeling the satisfaction of trying. The growing process does not require perfect outcomes to enjoy it.

Think of inner worth as a seed. Love is the fertilizer. When a seed starts to grow, we don't criticize it for not being a mature plant yet. Rather we put it in the sunlight, water and fertilize it, and enjoy watching it grow. When children begin to walk, we don't condemn them for falling, but clap for joy and encourage them further. Building self-esteem requires a similar approach.

While there are many strategies for building self-esteem, this one has been found to improve it within just a few weeks.

1. Think of your strengths for a moment (it is usually easier to identify weaknesses than strengths). For example, are you ever *reasonably* (circle those that apply to you): accepting, adventurous, brave, cheerful, composed, courteous, cooperative, creative, dependable, determined, disciplined, ethical, flexible, forgiving, fair, friendly, handy, industrious, kind, loyal, neat, open minded, organized, patient, persuasive, playful, punctual, respectful, self-accepting, self-controlled, thrifty, trusting, sincere, steady, or tactful? Are you *reasonably* good at (again, circle those that describe you): socializing, listening, cooking, sports, cleaning, working, befriending, singing, learning, leading, making decisions, following, helping,

encouraging, planning, listening to criticism, correcting mistakes, telling stories, being an example, enjoying life, budgeting, talking yourself out of a jam, entertaining yourself or others? Perfection was not required to circle these items, since *nobody* does any of these all of the time or perfectly. However, if you circled any of these and have managed to maintain reasonable sanity in a very complex world, give yourself a pat on the back. Then continue.

2. Write ten positive statements about yourself that are meaningful and realistic/true. You may develop the statements from the strengths you circled above, generate your own statements, or do both. Examples might be: "I am a loyal, responsible member of my _____(unit, family, etc.)"; "I am clean, orderly, etc."; "I am a concerned listener." If you mention a role that you perform well, try to add specific personal characteristics that explain why. For example, instead of saying only that one is a good unit member, one might write that he sizes up situations quickly and reacts decisively. Roles can change (e.g., after an injury or with age), but character and personality traits can be expressed across many different roles.

3. Find a place to relax undisturbed for 15-20 minutes. Meditate upon one statement and the evidences for its accuracy for a minute or two. Repeat this for each statement.

4. Repeat this exercise every day for at least a week. Each day, add an additional statement.

5. Several times each day, look at an item on the list, and for about two minutes meditate on the evidences for its accuracy.

If you prefer, you can write the statements on index cards and carry them with you. It is not unusual to hear people who try this strategy say, "At first I didn't believe these statements, but eventually I found myself singing on the way to work."

Realistic Optimism

Realistic optimism doesn't mean that you expect everything to turn out perfectly. Rather it is the attitude that if you try your best things are likely to turn out in the best possible way. It is also expecting that no matter how bad things get, you can still find something to enjoy and look forward to. Decades of research indicate that optimists are not only happier than pessimists, but are mentally healthier, more resistant to stress, more satisfied with their relationships, medically healthier, and they perform better in high-stress environments. Optimists are more likely to anticipate bad and good outcomes, plan accordingly, and persist in doing their best. They don't waste time getting bogged down in negativity.

When things go badly, pessimists typically explain it by thinking it's:
- *Personal* (e.g., due to something about me that's wrong, such as "I'm incompetent, an idiot.")
- *Pervasive* ("I mess up everything; My whole life stinks.")
- *Permanent* ("Things will never change. I might as well give up.")

In contrast, optimists explain bad events by thinking it's:
- *Not personal* ("This is a tough *situation*. I didn't *perform* well. Next time I'll try something different.")
- *Specific* ("I do well at other things. I had a bad day; that doesn't mean I mess up everything.")
- *Temporary* ("Things will probably improve. I'll learn and grow. Tomorrow will likely be better.")

Rather than giving up when the going gets tough, optimists also tend to see the silver lining. Like taking a military inventory, they look at adversity and see what's left to work with. For example, a wounded warrior thinks, "I lost a leg, but at least I didn't lose an eye. At least I didn't die. At least I can still enjoy music." Survivors' pride is reflected in comments like, "At least I realized I can survive almost anything. At least I realize what's most important in life. At least I still have my goals, my faith, and my sense of humor. At least I can still look forward to meeting good people." There is the humorous story of two neighbors who went through a divorce. One became dispirited and housebound. The other boldly stepped out the door, and confidently exclaimed, "Next!"

The optimist imagines a better life and makes goals to accomplish it. You might try this writing exercise: Describe a bright future, one in which you've worked hard and achieved the goals you most desire. Describe what you have done to reach those goals. Doing this for thirty minutes each day for four days has been found to improve mood.

Gratitude

Happy people regard life's good things with awe, appreciation, and wonder—or, in other words, gratitude. Gratitude counters the tendency to dwell on problems, increases our capacity to enjoy our lives, and improves brain chemistry. Gratitude builds relationships as we realize the good people have done for us, and reminds us that we don't need to own more stuff in order to enjoy life. Thus, warriors might look back on their service and dwell not on the hardships, but the good people they rubbed shoulders with, and the experiences and opportunities they had.

Keeping a gratitude journal has been found to increase happiness. Each night, for about five minutes, simply list five things you are grateful for over the previous twenty-four hours. Briefly describe in writing why you appreciate each—what it means, how it makes you feel, and why it happened. Do this for two weeks. Alternatively, pick one night a week, and list five things you are thankful for over the past week. Keep this up for six to ten weeks or longer. You might describe something that went well, something that was funny or pleasant, an accomplishment, things you learned, conveniences/comforts, a scene in nature, good medical care, or a good feeling. Either approach has been found to raise happiness. You might also express gratitude or appreciation to people for the good things they do—especially those you lead and your family. A letter of gratitude to someone who has touched your life benefits both the giver and the receiver.

Grateful reminiscing is an effective tool of resilient survivors. Try recalling pleasant memories in great detail. First, make a list of your favorite memories. Then recall one memory at a time, using all of your senses. Even the grateful processing of troubling memories can help to settle them. For example, after they've written about the difficult facts and feelings concerning a traumatic event, resilient survivors often find benefit in writing about the positive consequences that have resulted even from this bad situation (ways they've grown, recognizing strengths they didn't think they had, realizing what they most cherish, and making new goals and priorities in their lives).

Altruism

Altruism means that we are unselfishly concerned for the good of others; we wish to give another a leg up. Altruistic people are happier and more likely to succeed at work, in love, and at being healthy. In all age groups studied, doing good for others gives more pleasure than passive or recreational activities, such as watching TV or shopping. Try selecting one day a week for six weeks to do five acts of kindness. Do these cheerfully and without expectation of personal rewards. Kindnesses can be small (e.g., saying hello; saying, "Thanks for your good service"; giving a smile or a bigger tip) or larger (helping a buddy or neighbor without being asked, helping a child with homework, sending a thank you note to someone who made a difference, or volunteering for a good cause). Sometimes one can practice "guerilla kindness"—just look around and see what needs doing.

Humor

Humor, which is usually plentiful in the service, can lighten and lubricate life's darkest moments. Nearly all service members can recount at least one humorous tale that helped them endure even the worst times. Humor is the ability to amuse or be amused, to see the comical and find pleasure in any situation. Humor is bigger than jokes. It allows us to see even bad situations in a new light—with a sense of play, inner peace, and hope. Humor comes in many forms. In general, the most beneficial forms draw people together or laugh at life's comical aspects without putting anyone down. By contrast, aggressive or hostile humor makes people feel belittled. People generally like to be around people who have a wholesome sense of humor, and tend to avoid people who use humor as a hammer to constantly beat down others or themselves. Some helpful guidelines:

1. *Try noticing the joyful aspects of life before trying to be funny* (e.g., nature's beauty, things others do well). Dispense compliments at every honest opportunity, rather than criticism.

2. *Then simply chuckle at the incongruous, comical, amusing, ludicrous, or absurd.* Such situations are all around us. Simply be aware. If you bring others into the laughter, that's icing on the cake.

3. *Be kind and affectionate.* Ensure that humor builds bonds, not walls. Teasing for example, even when offered in a good-natured way, usually is more upsetting than the teaser realizes. Be especially cautious about sarcasm, hateful/aggressive humor, humor intended to dominate or demean, or laughing at outsiders (an exception is that POWs often bond together by secretly poking fun at powerful and cruel captors). Be sure that your humor isn't invalidating another's viewpoint or blocking another person's serious attempt to problem solve. Be especially cautious with humor directed at the insecure, anxious, depressed, guilty, or overly serious. If you are uncertain about how humor is being received, ask (e.g., "I was just trying to lighten things up. Was that OK?"). Then listen to the other person's response.

4. *Be yourself.* You needn't force humor. Use the humor type you are most comfortable with, whether that is telling a funny real-life story or joke or just enjoying a comical moment with a buddy or small group of friends.

5. *Know when not to be funny.* Not every moment needs to be turned into a joke. One who clowns around too much isn't taken seriously. While a light comment might help when someone is in pain, it can often backfire. If a loved one has a genuine concern, trying to make a joke of it can frustrate them.

6. *Use self-effacing humor sparingly.* A secure person can usually laugh at his/her own imperfections, and can put others at ease by doing so. However, don't overdo it. Putting oneself down too much can turn people off.

Moral Strength

Happy people behave in ways that promote peace of conscience and minimize regrets. When asked about what it was like to be a living saint, Mother Teresa in effect said, "Holiness is a simple duty for everyone in whatever position in life we are." Thus, one can be a holy teacher, parent, cop, or warrior. In nearly all cultures, the most valued moral strengths include courage, honesty, respect, responsibility, trustworthiness, fairness, benevolence, courtesy, and self-control. It may be the minority that chooses to live ethically, but we can choose to be part of that minority, realizing the long-term benefits of doing what is best for self and others. In a quiet moment, you might ask yourself if there is anything that disturbs your peace, damages your reputation with self, or leads others to distrust you. Without self-condemnation, rate how well you are living the character strengths just listed. Describe a time in the past when you demonstrated each of these strengths. Finally, describe what you could do to demonstrate each of these strengths better and more often. The standard is not perfection, but to be trying your personal best, and committing to improving every time you slip. Find satisfaction in all progress you make. Don't let discouragement take root.

Spirituality and Religion

Spirituality is the search for the sacred. For most this means striving to draw closer to God, to others, and to the highest values of humankind. Religion comes from the Latin word *religio,* meaning "to bind together," and suggests our attempts to connect to the sacred goals mentioned above.

The vast majority of studies document religion's positive effects, ranging from greater happiness and resilience to: greater optimism and altruism; better physical and mental health; more satisfaction with marriage and sex; and less substance use, divorce, suicide, guilt, and fear of death.

Researchers usually measure religion by *beliefs* (e.g., how important and comforting one's beliefs are; how much one tries to live them) and *practices* (attending worship services, praying or studying sacred writings at home, living ethically and charitably). In the research, it is not affiliation or denomination (e.g., whether one calls oneself Methodist, Jew, or Catholic) that predicts benefits of religion, but the degree to which people actually live their religion. Especially predictive of benefits are *attendance* (e.g., those who attend worship services weekly are far happier than those who attend rarely or not at all) and *religious certainty* (e.g., faith in God and the truth of one's beliefs, such as life after death).

Wholesome religion supports spirituality. Resilient survivors often cite religious faith as critical to their survival. Most Americans believe in God, consider religion important, and think they are religious, or spiritual, or both.

Religion only correlates with unhappiness when one has an unhappy image of God. In several studies those who regard God as kind and caring are happier than those who regard God as punitive, unresponsive, and unloving. Spiritual confusion or ambivalence can also be unsettling. For example, holding, but not living by beliefs, can undermine spiritual security. On average, agnostics are less happy than atheists, who are less happy than believers.

Pathways to spirituality include:

1. *Treat mental disorders, such as PTSD, depression, and anxiety.* These can numb spiritual feelings.

2. *Actively participate in religious practices for intrinsic reasons*, not external rewards, such as social standing, career success, or praise. Greater benefits accrue for those who practice for inner reasons with full commitment.

3. *Consider releasing unworkable spiritual assumptions*, such as:

   - *If God really loved me, God wouldn't let me suffer. God doesn't care.* Job, Peter, and Jesus, to name a few, suffered greatly. Does that mean they weren't loved? Suffering is not necessarily an indication of divine disfavor, just as comfort does not necessarily indicate divine favor. Suffering is part of life. It can ultimately deepen compassion, be a means for growth, and stimulate our most meaningful work in a way that comfort will not.

   - *God should ensure that only good happens.* This can keep us stuck in anger and blame. In an imperfect world where people have free choice, bad sometimes happens—sometimes through the fault of others, sometimes through our own fault, and sometimes randomly. An alternative thought might consider that the ultimate purpose in adversity might not be immediately obvious. Sometimes we create the meaning in adversity by our responses to it.

   - *God won't forgive me for that.* Where is that written? Bouncing back from mistakes and starting anew is one important form of spiritual resilience. *Everyone* has the right to try again.

   - *I must forget my troubling past.* That isn't possible. Instead, the spiritual warrior can bring it to God, the master healer. It is then possible to remember the past, but without feeling the emotional distress.

   - *Religion and being good will protect me from adversity.* These won't necessarily, but they *can* provide the inner peace and strength needed to meet adversity without hatred or bitterness.

52

4. *Don't be surprised if faith initially weakens after the war zone experience.* Spiritual growth isn't simple, nor is it necessarily linear. Although adversity can deepen one's faith, about 30% of people experience a weakening of faith after trauma. Initially one might feel numb, angry, or spiritually adrift. With time—especially if one turns toward rather than away from spirituality and religious practice—faith can deepen.

5. *Don't be surprised by initial discomfort in trying to practice religiously.* In the war zone, sometimes warriors feel as if "God isn't here." All congregants might not be understanding or welcoming to returning warriors. Don't let these discourage you. Allow time to readjust. Remember that you have as much right to be a part of a religious community as anyone else. After all, you've defended one of the four great freedoms—freedom of worship.

Money: Attitudes and Management

Although the amount of money or possessions one has doesn't affect happiness much, the ways we view and manage money do affect happiness. Research suggests that the following steps might increase happiness:

1. *Spend money on memories, rather than material objects.* Instead of things, such as jewelry or clothes, consider spending on a vacation, concert, trip, or meal.

2. *Spend some money to help make others happy*—gifts, donations, and making memories for others.

3. *Budget wisely.* Happy people tend to live by a written budget and live within their means. They also tend to pay bills as they come in, have wills, and purchase insurance (life, disability, etc.). Peace of mind tends to come from a sense of control over our resources, not necessarily the amount of wealth we possess.

4. *Save 5-10% of your income.* Savings give a secure feeling.

5. *Avoid debt as much as possible.* Interest on loans accrues constantly, even when we sleep or vacation. Avoid using credit cards for luxuries or extravagant purchases, and only use them when you have sufficient cash to cover the purchase. Beyond a modest home or car, or needed education, try to avoid debt.

6. *When you think about money, try not to compare yourself to other people.* Wealth does not change one's intrinsic worth. Think of how you contribute, not the size of your paycheck.

7. *Live simply and be content with what you have.* In terms of comforts and conveniences, like running water and heating, the average American lives like royalty compared to those living 100 years ago. Many of the things that bring contentment cost little or nothing. Conversely, the pursuit of wealth can deprive us of the time we need to enjoy life's simple pleasures—like sunsets or reading a good book.

Meaning and Purpose

People who sense that their lives have meaning and purpose are happier and more resilient. For example, WWII concentration camp survivor Viktor Frankl observed that those who had something to live for withstood their suffering better. He wrote that people must discover their own unique ways to make their lives worthwhile and significant. In general, he wrote, people do this by giving something meaningful to the world (e.g., establishing, joining, or contributing to a worthy cause; creating something useful or beautiful); developing and using personal strengths (e.g., goodness of character, compassion, altruism, etc.); and experiencing and enjoying life's wholesome pleasures/beauties (e.g., nature, intimate love, friends, recreation, improving the mind through education). Many people find meaning and purpose through their work. Ideally, people find jobs or careers they love. Others find ways to redefine their jobs. For example, some happy hospital cleaning staff members view their work as a calling that helps patients heal and the medical staff work more effectively. They go beyond their required cleaning duties and try to beautify rooms, say, by adding flowers and bringing smiles to patients. Each job can be meaningful. In WWII, General Patton told his truck drivers that without them the war would be lost. Consider how your work might benefit yourself and others.

Social Intelligence

People skills help us love, lead, lift, motivate, persuade, get along with, respond to, and ask for help of others. People with social intelligence generally fare better in all areas of life, while those lacking people skills tend to derail careers and relationships. Socially intelligent people tend to be likeable, respectful, believable, genuine, positive, approachable, appreciative, interested, and enthused. They tend to listen more than they speak. Importantly, they empathize—that is, they sense or attune to another's emotions and thoughts in a caring way.

Socially intelligent leaders build others up—helping them to be confident and to do their best work without fear of failing. They communicate expectations clearly and calmly, and praise good work. They are perceived as being "in the trenches" with their people, and caring about them as individuals.

Socially intelligent people apply people skills at home. Some helpful ideas:

1. *Success in marriage usually takes time.* It typically takes 10-15 years for a couple to reach high quality intimacy: At first couples romantically think that their partner is perfect, able to fulfill all their needs. Over time, couples recognize differences in their partners, and struggle to work out these differences. Eventually, they choose to stay together, cooperate, and interdepend because they enjoy being a team. Note that the prospects of marital satisfaction are good. Among those who describe their marriages as very unhappy, 80% of those who stick it out for five years will say that their marriage is happy. The likelihood of success is better if partners learn good couples skills, such as how to disagree in ways that strengthen relationships (see the resources at the end of this booklet).

2. *Rather than getting defensive or trying to quickly fix a problem, first try to simply validate your partner's feelings and viewpoints.* If your partner is upset, sit down, face him/her, and calmly say, "Tell me about it." Try to acknowledge the other person's feelings, saying something like, "I can see how that would be upsetting. Tell me more to help me understand." Check out your understanding by restating ("It sounds like you are feeling X, because of Y. Is that right?"). Don't mind-read or speak for your partner. Simply restate what your partner has said. When your partner feels *completely* heard and understood, only then express how you see the issue. It might take several hours of calm back-and-forth discussion for both partners to feel understood. When you arrive at this point, then set a time to brainstorm and try to solve the problem. This approach takes work and time but, especially for hot issues, the effort is worthwhile.

3. *Accentuate the positives.* Appreciate, don't criticize. Criticizing creates resentment, and is a difficult habit to reverse. Structure time for fun and friendship—time that is free of talking about problems. Brainstorm fun activities, and then alternate from each other's list. If you have a concern or criticism, make sure compliments and positive encounters outweigh these by at least five to one.

4. *Have a weekly couple's meetings to anticipate possible problems, plan, and value the partner.* Emphasize what is going well. Thank your partner for what he/she is doing well.

5. *Put your spouse first.* Greet your spouse cheerfully. Remember the courtesies that you used when courting, such as saying *please* and *thank you.*

6. *Be 100% honest and faithful.* These strengths characterize happy couples.

7. *Hold weekly family nights.* Their purpose is to create family bonds and memories. Anything that is fun works: games, picnics, discussions, gardening, planning a vacation, or learning together.

8. *Hold regular family councils to coordinate calendars, share goals, go over chores, plan, and encourage.* The environment is open, safe, and positive. If a child wishes to change or improve a family routine, they must suggest a possible solution to discuss.
9. *Follow up family meetings with regular mom or dad interviews with each child.* Tell the child, "This is a time for you to talk about your interests and concerns, accomplishments, goals, and so forth. What would you like to talk about?" Be sure to mostly listen, and then express appreciation.
10. *Correct children in private.*
11. *Tap the power of family dinners.* In families that eat together, all members of the family benefit in many ways. Make dinner together a priority. Turn off distracting electronics.

Balance and Fun

Resilient warriors keep their life in balance so that if one area isn't going well another area can provide satisfaction. They also derive enjoyment from a wide range of activities.

Wholesome, pleasant activities help to keep the brain sharp and the mood upbeat, and appear to improve work performance. Often, when people get too busy or stressed, they jettison pleasant activities to save time. This tends to depress the mood. As this happens, they start to assume that nothing could lift the mood again, so they stop engaging in the very activities that would make them feel better. So the mood slips further. To counter this downward spiral, consider all the things that have ever been pleasant to do. To prime your memory, consider the list below.

- Being with pleasant people, friends, family, or service buddies
- Meeting someone new
- Going to a restaurant, club, or tavern
- Being at celebrations (birthdays, weddings, parties, get-togethers, etc.)
- Having an honest discussion
- Amusing others, making another person laugh or smile
- Playing with children, telling a child a story, holding or watching a sleeping child
- Doing a challenging job well
- Learning something new (e.g., new hobby, language, or skill)
- Repairing something (e.g., fixing a car or bike)
- Doing volunteer work
- Having a good meal
- Fishing, hunting, woodworking, photography, gardening, collecting things, or some other hobby
- Dressing up
- Going to bed early, sleeping soundly, and awakening refreshed
- Wearing jeans or other comfortable clothes
- Going to a concert
- Playing sports
- Taking a trip or vacation
- Reading a good book
- Being outdoors (beach, country, mountains, kicking leaves, walking in the sand, floating in lakes, camping, boating, going on a picnic)
- Biking
- Beautifying or fixing up my home/quarters
- Going to a sports event
- Playing or singing music

- Thinking about something good in the future; making goals and plans
- Taking a warm bath
- Being around animals or pets
- Taking a nap
- Listening to nature sounds (rain, wind, waves) or feeling a breeze on my skin
- Getting or giving a backrub
- Reminiscing with old friends
- Sitting and thinking
- Driving through the country with the windows open or the top down
- Being physically close to someone I love
- Watching a good movie

Make a plan to do several of these, especially those that have been pleasant in the past or that you think you would enjoy. Write them down on your calendar. Then do them. Start small and with the simplest activities. Set yourself up to find pleasure in the activity (e.g., "I will enjoy the sunshine, the breeze, talking, etc."). You might want to turn off the electronic devices in order to be fully receptive to the experience. Be satisfied with partial success—if you find even some pleasure, consider the activity successful.

Eight

Advanced Warrior Skills: Meditation

It's a perfect combination of aggressive action taking place in an atmosphere of total tranquility...just totally peaceful.
Billie Jean King

Meditation may be thought of as experiencing our true, happy nature. It is not surprising, then, that adding meditation to happiness training gives an added boost in happiness, while giving additional reductions in anxiety and depression. In fact, meditating has been found to confer many other beneficial effects, including improved cognitive abilities, situational awareness, medical health, and heart coherence. In this chapter we'll explore two methods of meditating that are particularly effective for warriors before, during, and after deployment: mindfulness mediation and integral yoga meditation.

Mindfulness Meditation

If time for resilience training were severely limited, many warriors say that mindfulness meditation is the one skill they would learn. It is that effective. Since being introduced into Western medical circles in 1979, researchers have concluded that mindfulness:

- Increases positive and decreases negative emotions, affecting the activity in various regions of the brain that are associated with mood
- Increases resilience and the ability to cope with stress
- Improves reaction time, productivity, empathy, relationship satisfaction, inner security, vitality, and sleep quality
- Enlarges various regions of the brain, including the hippocampus and prefrontal cortex
- Improves the ability to pay attention; synchronizes various brain regions involved in cognitive functions
- Boosts immune function; reduces chronic pain, blood pressure, psoriasis, and a wide range of other medical symptoms
- Reduces impulsivity and reactivity to criticism, conflict, and other stressors (even torture)
- Increases comfort with adversity and stress symptoms

Mindfulness changes the way we *respond* to our environment without attempting to change the outer world—or even our thoughts. Instead of *fighting* with what is, or *reacting* with strong emotions, mindfulness practice teaches us to be fully aware of each moment with calm, compassion, and equanimity. Eventually, mindfulness helps us to experience even the strongest, most distressing emotions, thoughts, and bodily discomforts calmly and without undue distress. This is why mindfulness training is often included in PTSD treatments for warriors.

Mindfulness derives from Eastern teachings. However, the practice of mindfulness readily harmonizes with nearly any tradition imaginable.

In the Eastern view, each person is of two minds, the wisdom mind and the ordinary mind. Visualize two concentric circles, as in the figure on the next page. At the center is our wisdom mind, or true happy nature—who we truly are. The wisdom mind is happy, wise, compassionate, good humored, dignified, humble, hopeful, whole, peaceful, and fully aware. When we are grounded in our wisdom mind, we respond to the world in the most effective way. Problems arise, however, when we are pulled away from our wisdom mind into the ordinary mind. The ordinary mind is characterized by swirling, effortful, and scattered thoughts. The ordinary mind endlessly thinks, plans, worries, regrets, obsesses, judges, avoids, hurries, dramatizes, and fights against the way life is—resulting in emotional and physical distress. You've undoubtedly heard the expression that someone is beside himself/herself with worry, anger, or other strong negative emotions. This means they are separated from the wisdom mind and stuck in the ordinary mind. Racing thoughts actually distract us and block our ability to focus. The ordinary mind covers the wisdom mind and causes most of our suffering. It attaches to things that are not necessary for our happiness, such as pride, jealousy, or material goods. So the idea of meditation is to get underneath the ordinary mind, grounded in the peaceful wisdom mind. Mindfulness is not a way of thinking; it is a way of being.

THE NATURE OF MIND

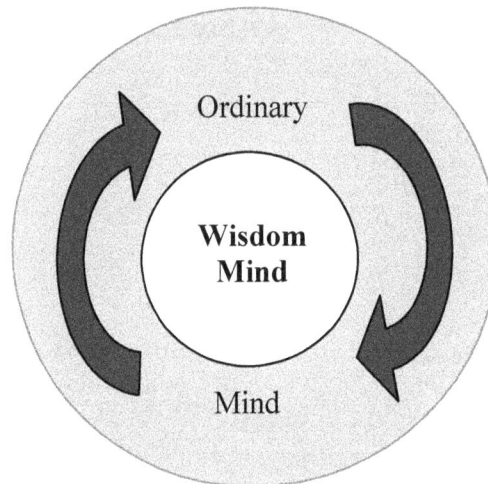

In Eastern teaching, the word for mind also means heart. Mindfulness is about connecting with the innate attitudes of the heart. We shall highlight seven of these attitudes.

- *Compassion* is the most important attitude. Compassion is often translated as gentle friendliness or loving kindness. Compassion means feeling sorrow and empathy for suffering and the desire to help. Eastern masters, however, teach that it is as important to feel compassion for oneself as it is to feel compassion for others. When we respond to stressors with compassion we are calmer and happier. When we are calmer and happier, we can respond more effectively to daily challenges.

- *Vastness.* The wisdom mind is broad and deep, large enough to embrace any stressor compassionately. The wisdom mind is often likened to a vast ocean. At its depths the ocean is calm. Looking from the calm depths, we view stressors as waves at the surface. The waves swell, and then are absorbed into the vast deep ocean, leaving the inner depths unchanged. This perspective reminds us that the surface can constantly change, but our center has all the resources needed to fully face whatever storms arise confidently and calmly. (In treating PTSD, for example, mindfulness teaches that one is not broken, only stuck in the fragmented ordinary mind. The goal is to rest in the vast wholeness of the wisdom mind.)

- *Acceptance.* To accept is to see with full awareness what is, without judging, criticizing, or over-thinking the situation. When we accept, we simply notice, without trying to fix, change, or escape the situation. That is, we first bring compassionate awareness to the situation, so that the appropriate response will become apparent. Notice that acceptance does not mean passive resignation. It simply means that we fully take in the situation before we do anything. This stance has important implications. Often people experience strong anger (an ordinary-mind reaction) when they are really afraid to face fear or pain. They might drink to escape these feelings, but drinking doesn't change them. Mindfulness teaches us to simply acknowledge the fear and pain without judgment—to gently turn *toward* our experience. Compassion eventually soothes those distressing emotions. We greet them cordially, watch them rise like the waves,

58

and eventually be absorbed into the ocean. In day-to-day living, acceptance teaches us to first see clearly the way it is, not the way the ordinary mind says it is, before attempting to solve, fix, or change the problem. Acceptance is the primary response. Sometimes it is the only response needed. Paradoxically, acceptance is associated with effective planning and action, whereas avoidance keeps us stuck.

- *Non-attachment*. Attachment is the root of unhappiness. We lock on to the thought that "I must have something to be happy." That something might be a material possession, such as a car. Then we push ourselves feverishly to obtain that car, and feel sad if we don't get it. If we get it, we worry that something might happen to it, or get angry if someone scratches it. Or, we could be attached to status, appearances, prestige, a relationship, or even happiness. Attachments keep us tense and battling in the ordinary mind. When we release the attachment and allow ourselves to come home to the wisdom mind, we realize that we already have within what is needed to be happy. Notice that we can still actively pursue what we value. However, in mindfulness practice we release the vice-like grip and don't strive for anything in the moment. Later, if we choose to, we can act with greater relaxation, clarity, and efficiency.
- *Beginner's mind*. The expert learns little. The child who is fully open usually learns more. In mindfulness we do not prematurely foreclose our experience with preconceived judgments or expectations, such as "I can't meditate", "I'll never improve", or "I must do this just right." We simply practice with an open, flexible mind, being neither overly optimistic nor cynically pessimistic. We just allow the experience to unfold and notice what happens, without trying to make anything happen.
- *Equanimity*. We greet whatever we experience, whether positive or negative, with the same calm response. In mindfulness, both positive and negative emotions are considered important, and each is greeted in the same calm, non-judgmental, unattached way.
- *Commitment*. Those who practice mindfulness meditation usually find that starting with twenty minutes per day, and progressing to 45 minutes per day or longer, six days a week, is most effective. Practice even if you don't feel like it; the beneficial effects of practice accumulate over time. As with exercise, any practice is better than none.

Jon Kabat-Zinn, Ph.D., introduced mindfulness meditation to Western medical circles at the University of Massachusetts Medical School. His eight-week training program is called Mindfulness-based Stress Reduction, which we will overview here in abbreviated and somewhat modified form.[xii] It all starts with the humble raisin. Practice each exercise in sequence, since each builds on the one before it.

Exercise: The Raisins

The purpose of this exercise is to eat two raisins mindfully with full awareness over a ten- to fifteen-minute period.

1. Hold two raisins gently in the palm of your hand with a curious, good-humored attitude.
2. Pick one up and notice all the details of the raisin—the ridges, stem, translucence, color, and aroma. Notice the sensations in your fingers as you feel the surface of the raisin. Roll it between your fingers next to your ear and notice what that sounds like.
3. Notice your body as you hold it, noticing tension as you move it slowly toward your mouth. Sense the air against your skin as your hand moves slowly, much as you'd feel the water against your hand in the bath. Notice whether your body is signaling hunger. Pay attention to all the sensations in your hand and moving arm.

[xii] The ensuing sections on mindfulness are adapted from Schiraldi, G. R. (2007), *Ten Simple Solutions for Building Self-Esteem*, Oakland, CA: New Harbinger.

4. As you get ready to put it in your mouth, you might notice yourself thinking things like "I like (dislike) raisins. Mom used to give them to us for snacks. I'd like to eat lunch. I really don't have time to do this raisin exercise. There are probably a lot of calories in this raisin. What's this got to do with resilience?" This is good. Each time such thoughts arise, greet them cordially (thinking is what the ordinary mind does), and simply bring back your attention to eating the raisin.
5. Notice how your mouth accepts the raisin. As you let the raisin sit on your tongue, just sense it there and notice what it feels like before eating it. After a while place it on different areas of the tongue. Notice whether you salivate and taste the raisin.
6. Take a single bite and notice the flavor. You might notice a burst of flavor that is more intense than it seems when you mindlessly eat raisins.
7. Chew slowly, paying attention to what that is like, and then notice the intent to swallow. As you swallow, follow the raisin down into your stomach. Notice the aftertaste and sensations in your body.
8. When you finish, do it again with the second raisin, being fully and calmly present for the experience.

Most of the elements of mindfulness are introduced in this exercise: being calmly present for an experience moment by moment without judging or emotionally reacting; being aware of the wandering mind, and gently escorting it back to the moment without judging; the beginner's mind (even though you might think all raisins are the same, eating the second raisin is not the same experience as eating the first); and realizing how much of life we miss when we are not mindful. Many people notice that the experience of eating a raisin is more intense when the mind is focused on the present moment, and that they really notice flavors that they miss when they are in a hurry. Some say that they'd probably eat less if they were mindful because they'd enjoy each bite more and would notice when hunger signals had stopped. Warriors observe that this exercise teaches calm situational awareness.

Exercise: Mindful Breathing

This is a very effective meditation practice that helps us learn to be more peaceful in our own bodies, and to get under the racing thoughts in our heads. It takes about ten to fifteen minutes. Practice it once a day for a week.
1. Sit comfortably in the meditator's posture: Feet are flat on the floor; hands are resting, unfolded, comfortably in the lap, with palms up or down. The back is comfortably erect. Imagine that the spine is aligned like a column of golden coins resting one atop the other. The head is neither forward nor back; the chin is neither up nor down. The torso is held with dignity and grace, like a majestic mountain. The mountain is constant and secure, despite the clouds that cover it or the storms that batter it.
2. Allow your eyes to close. Release tension in the shoulders, neck, and jaw. Let the abdomen be soft and relaxed. Permit your body to relax and settle. Let yourself begin to settle in the wisdom mind.
3. Gently and with good humor be aware for a moment of the attitudes of mindfulness that already exist within, such as compassion, vastness, acceptance, and nonattachment. In this meditation, you are not striving to make anything in particular happen. Just notice what occurs.
4. Let awareness go to your breathing, as you breathe abdominally (allow your upper body to be relaxed and still; the only movement is your abdomen rising as you breathe in and falling as you breathe out). Notice your breathing, as you would watch waves flow in and out from the shore on the beach. As your breath is flowing, sense the parts of your body that are moving. You might sense the rising and stretching in your abdomen as you breathe in. You might notice the breath moving through your nostrils and throat and in and out of your lungs. Perhaps you

notice your heart beating, slightly faster on the in-breath and slightly slower on the out-breath. Each breath is different, so pay attention to the entire breath with the beginner's mind.

5. As you breathe, thoughts will come and go. To fight them is to increase tension, so simply notice your mind wandering, and each time you notice that it has wandered, gently bring it back to focusing on the breath. The object is not to stop yourself from thinking. Rather, it is to feel satisfaction each time you notice your mind wandering. This is what the ordinary mind does. Congratulate yourself each time you mindfully notice this, and gently, kindly, patiently return your awareness to the breath without judging. Think of this as practice in responding to life with loving kindness.

6. Release, relax, and rest in the breath. Notice fully each part of the in-breath, the out-breath, and each subtle changing moment. Rest your mind in your belly, sensing what this is like.

7. And now feel the breath as if it were a wave that filled the entire body. Underneath the breath notice a deeper calm, a peace within.

8. When you are finished notice how you feel. Let that feeling go, just as you let awareness of the breath come and go.

Exercise: Body Scan

We feel emotions and physical sensations in the body. Yet we often try to manage these in the head. We might think, "Oh, no. I don't want to feel that emotion. Not again. I've got to stop feeling that." Or, "This pain is terrible; I've got to find a way to kill it." The more we fight the feelings and sensations, the more we suffer. We are often quite out of touch with the body as we live in our heads—being more connected to television, computers, or cell phones than to our bodies. We might be obsessed with the image of our body in the mirror without being in tune with our body, just as we may eat without really tasting. The body scan meditation will prepare us to eventually experience emotional and physical discomfort with kindness and calmness, without trying to push it away, run from it, or think ourselves out of it. This meditation teaches us to simply welcome in each sensation. We watch it kindly and dispassionately, and then let our awareness of the sensation dissolve. As we simply watch sensations, we notice that they often change; they come and go. When we do not tense up, but instead relax into the sensation, our *response* to the sensation changes. Many people observe that they feel grounded when they are centered in their bodies instead of their heads—peacefully observing the comings and goings of bodily sensations, and holding whatever comes up in calm awareness. The idea in this meditation is not to *think about* each region of the body, but to place your awareness deep inside it, feeling from inside. Practice this meditation for about forty minutes daily, for at least a week.

1. Lie down on your back in a place where you are unlikely to be disturbed. Close your eyes. Remember especially the attitudes of loving kindness, acceptance, non-judgment, letting go, and good humor.

2. Breathe and let your mind settle; let your mind rest calmly in your body.

3. Notice how your body as a whole feels at this moment without judging. Feel your skin against the ground or bed. Notice the temperature of the air around you and how it feels. Be aware of how your body feels—is it comfortable, or is there any tension, pain, or itching? Notice the intensity of these sensations and whether they change or stay the same.

4. In a moment you will breathe in and out of one region of your body several times, paying full attention to all the sensations that you experience. It is as though your mind is resting in that area of the body. Then when you are ready, you will release your awareness, letting awareness of that region dissolve as you also release tension in that area. Next you'll bring your awareness in a similar way to the next region. Each time your mind wanders, gently bring it back to the region on which you are focusing without judging. Let's begin. We'll give directions starting with the toes of your left foot. Then we'll progress in a similar fashion to the other regions of the body.

5. Bring kind, openhearted attention to the toes of your left foot, letting your mind rest there. Imagine that you are breathing in and out of your toes. Perhaps you imagine air from your in-breath flowing down through your nose, lungs, abdomen, and legs into your toes, and then, with your out-breath, out from your toes, up through your body, and though your nose. Allow yourself to feel any and all sensations in the toes—pressure from a sock, temperature, blood flow, pulsing, relaxation, tension, and so on. Notice any changes in these sensations as you breathe. If you feel nothing that is okay. Just notice whatever there is to experience without commenting or judging. When you are ready to leave this region, take a deeper and more intentional breath, following the breath down the toes once again. As you exhale, let awareness of the toes dissolve, releasing any tension or discomfort your body is willing to release at this time, as you bring awareness to the next region of your body (your left sole). Let your awareness stay in the next region in the same way for several breaths before moving on. As thoughts arise, silently and without judgment say, "Thinking, thinking." Gently return your awareness to the region of the body and your breathing. Approach each region with the beginner's mind, as though you've never before paid attention to that region. Watch whatever you experience without tensing or judging, but with kind, gentle, softhearted awareness. Repeat the process for each body part, following the list below.

- Left sole
- Left heel
- Top of left foot
- Left ankle
- Left shin and calf
- Left knee
- Left thigh
- Left side of groin
- Left hip
- Toes of right foot
- Right sole
- Right heel
- Top of right foot
- Right ankle
- Right shin and calf
- Right knee
- Right thigh
- Right side of groin
- Right hip
- Pelvic region, genitals, and buttocks
- Lower back
- Upper back
- Spinal column
- Stomach
- Chest
- Ribs
- Heart
- Lungs
- Shoulder blades
- Collar bones

- Shoulders
- Fingers of left hand
- Left palm
- Back of left hand
- Left wrist
- Left forearm
- Left elbow
- Left upper arm
- Left armpit
- Fingers of right hand
- Right palm
- Back of right hand
- Right wrist
- Right forearm
- Right elbow
- Right upper arm
- Right armpit
- Neck and throat (notice air flow)
- Nose (notice air flow and smells without judgment)
- Left ear
- Right ear
- Eyes
- Cheeks
- Forehead
- Temples
- Jaw and mouth
- Face
- Crown of head

6. Now be aware of your whole body, breathing in peaceful stillness. Go beneath your thoughts and feel the wholeness of the body. Notice what is moving or changing. Breathe through imaginary air holes in your head and feet. Breathe in through the head, following the breath down to the stomach, and, on the out-breath, follow the breath down the legs and out the toes. Then breathe in through the feet, following the in-breath to the stomach, and breathe out through the head. Ultimately feel the entire body breathing, like waves on the surface of the ocean, as you watch from the calm and peaceful depths.

Exercise: Smile Meditation

This beautiful meditation reminds us that happiness already exists within us as part of our true, happy nature. It is good to practice this at the beginning of the day, and throughout the day. Allow about ten to fifteen minutes for this meditation.

1. Assume the meditator's posture, sitting comfortably erect, with feet flat on the floor, and hands resting comfortably in the lap. The spine is straight like a stack of golden coins. The upper body is relaxed but erect, sitting in graceful dignity like a majestic mountain. Allow your eyes to close. Let your breathing help you settle into your restful wisdom mind.

2. Be aware of the playful, good-humored aspects of your true happy nature, or wisdom mind. Imagine for a moment what it would be like to smile. Perhaps you notice that just the idea of a

smile tends to evoke feelings of being content, happy, relaxed, and softhearted. Just the thought of smiling relaxes and softens your face.

3. Now allow a half smile to form on your face—perhaps a little twinkle that causes your eyes to sparkle, relaxing your face and jaw. The smile spreads across your face—bathing, soothing, and comforting your face.

4. Imagine that the happy feeling of your smile spreads to the neck and throat. Just sense happiness in that region, letting your mind rest there.

5. Now let happiness spread to the lungs, sensing the comfort it brings to that area. Perhaps happiness feels like a warm light there. Whatever it is, just accept that and allow it to be.

6. Now, let that feeling of happiness fill the heart, warming, and soothing it. Breathe and let the mind rest there. Just allow happiness to settle in your heart.

7. Let the happy feeling of that smile spread to the stomach and any other areas of the body in turn that you wish to focus on. Just sense the happiness in each region of the body.

8. Hold any thoughts that arise in kind friendliness, and return to experiencing the smile and happiness in the body. Conclude by sensing your whole body breathing and being comforted by the soothing, happy feeling of a smile.

Exercise: Sitting with Emotions

The meditation skills explained earlier in this chapter have prepared you for the following very powerful method of calming distressing emotions, and thereby taking care of yourself. This meditation teaches us to be calm and non-reactive in the presence of whatever emotions arise, good or bad.

In our Western culture, we are taught to flee or cover pain with painkillers, work, shopping, risky behaviors, or other forms of sedation that do not address the pain. We might take stimulants, instead of listening to our bodies and then "taking sleep" when tired. This meditation teaches us to turn gently toward pain with kind awareness. Softening our response changes the way we experience pain.

The wisdom mind is indeed vast, loving, and accepting—wide and deep enough to hold any distressing emotion. Thus, we can be open to whatever exists, penetrating distressing emotions with healing loving kindness. Instead of fighting thoughts, memories, and feelings, we can learn to just embrace them, remembering compassion. It is like sitting with your beloved who is in pain, listening, and saying: "Tell me about it. Whatever it is, it's okay." We listen without judging until the pain subsides and/or the person changes his response to the pain—relaxing, rather than fighting the pain.

In this meditation, we learn to watch distressing emotions from the vast, detached perspective of the wisdom mind. The pain is impersonal; we don't identify with the pain. We think, "There is pain," rather than "I have pain" or "I am the pain." Remembering that the ordinary mind creates much suffering as we resist pain ("Why do I have to suffer? It's not fair! I can't stand this pain!"), we change our response to pain by allowing the pain in. However, instead of bracing and tensing as we fight it, we relax into the pain with full acceptance. We don't judge emotions as bad or good; instead, we accept both with equanimity, allowing love to penetrate and dissolve the pain. It is recommended that this meditation be practiced for thirty minutes or more each day for at least a week.

1. Assume the meditator's posture, sitting comfortably erect, with feet flat on the floor, and hands resting comfortably in the lap. The spine is straight like a stack of golden coins. The upper body is relaxed but erect, sitting in graceful dignity like a majestic mountain. Allow your eyes to close. Let your breathing help you to settle into your peaceful wisdom mind.

2. Remember the key attitudes of acceptance, compassion, and vastness. Remember that you are already whole. Use the beginner's mind as you explore a new way to experience feelings.

3. Be aware of your breathing for several minutes. Let your belly be soft and relaxed, watching it rise and fall as you breathe in and out, becoming still, peaceful, settled, grounded, and really present.

4. Be aware of any feeling in your body, any sensation as it comes and goes, without judging or trying to change it.
5. Whenever you find your mind wandering, congratulate yourself for noticing this. Remember that thoughts are just thoughts, and not who you are, and bring your awareness gently back to breathing and sensing your body.
6. Recall a difficult situation, perhaps involving work or a relationship—and the feelings of unworthiness, inadequacy, sadness, worry about the future, or any other feelings that arise. Make a space for this situation. Give deep attention to these feelings. *Whatever* you are feeling is alright. Greet these feelings cordially, as you would greet an old friend.
7. Notice where in the body you feel the feelings (your stomach, chest, or throat, for example). Let yourself feel the feelings completely, with full acceptance. Don't think, "I'll tighten up and let these feelings in for a minute in order to get rid of them." This is not full acceptance. Rather, create a space that allows the feelings to be completely accepted.
8. Breathe into that region of the body with great love, as if fresh air and sunlight were entering a long-ignored and darkened room. Follow your breath all the way down through the nose, throat, lungs, and then to the part of the body where you sense the distressing emotion(s). Then follow the breath out of your body, until you find yourself settling. You might think of a kind, loving, accepting smile as you do this. Don't try to change or push the discomfort away. Don't brace or struggle with it. Just embrace it without judging it—with real acceptance, deep attention, loving kindness, and peace. Let the body soften and open around that area. The wisdom mind is vast enough to hold these feelings with great compassion; love is big enough to embrace, welcome, and penetrate the discomfort. Let your breath caress and soothe the feelings as you would your adored sleeping baby.
9. View the discomfort from the dispassionate perspective of the wisdom mind. It is as if you are watching waves of discomfort rise on the surface of the ocean, and then be reabsorbed into the vast ocean. The waves come and go without changing the basic nature of the ocean. If you find it helpful, you might think of loved ones who remind you of loving kindness—and let that loving kindness penetrate your awareness as you remember that difficult situation. Simply notice what happens to the feelings without trying to make them change.
10. When you are ready, take a deeper breath into that area of the body and, as you exhale, widen your focus to your body as a whole. Pay attention to your whole body's breathing, being aware of the wholeness and the vast, unlimited compassion of the wisdom mind that will hold any pain that comes and goes. Your attention now expands to the sounds you are hearing, just bringing them into awareness without commenting or judging. Simply listen with a half smile. Feel the air against your body; sense your whole body breathing. Notice all that you are aware of with a soft and open heart.
11. To conclude, say the following intentions silently to yourself: "May I remember loving kindness. May I be happy. May I be whole."

Exercise: Mindfulness-Based Cognitive Therapy

From calm thinking (see chapter 3) we learned a useful way for dealing with the drama that plays out in the ordinary mind: we first become aware of our distorted automatic thoughts and then replace these with more constructive thoughts. This tends to reduce the severity of the disturbing emotions that we experience. Further relief can be gained by becoming aware of, and replacing, our inaccurate core beliefs.

In Eastern psychology, automatic thoughts and core beliefs are just thoughts in the ordinary mind that do not reflect the deeper wisdom mind. In fact, trying to fight thinking with thinking can keep one locked in a tense struggle in the ordinary mind. Logic alone may not sufficiently soothe hurt feelings. Mindfulness offers an alternative to fighting thoughts with thinking. In mindfulness, we simply bring compassionate awareness to our thoughts, breathe into them, allow awareness of them to dissolve, and return to resting in the wisdom mind. The neural pathways associated with these negative thoughts degrade through disuse, as we fail to react emotionally to them and instead strengthen the pathways associated with the wisdom mind.

Return to chapter 3. Identify an emotionally charged automatic thought or core belief (e.g., "I'm out of control"). Instead of trying to change it, try sitting with it as follows:

1. Sit comfortably in the meditator's posture, breathing softly, resting in the wisdom mind.
2. Bring the thought into kind awareness without judging the thought. Notice where you sense the thought and associated feeling in your body and breathe into that area with loving kindness and complete acceptance.
3. Occasionally, if it is helpful, mindfully remind yourself:
   - It's just a thought.
   - Holding that thought in kind awareness.
   - Feeling compassion.
4. Keep breathing into the area of the body where you sense the thought until you are ready to release awareness of that thought.
5. With a deeper, more intentional breath, let awareness of that area dissolve as you become aware of your environment. Or, you might shift to a smile meditation.

Everyday Mindfulness

We can practice mindfulness in our everyday moments. Practice a smile meditation. Then choose an everyday activity to do mindfully. That is, fully experience the activity without getting caught up in judging, criticizing, or over-thinking. Simply bring kind awareness and acceptance to each moment. If you notice yourself being distracted by a thought, just escort your awareness back to the activity. For example, you might mindfully:

- Wake up
- Savor a meal (when eating, just eat—notice aromas, textures, tastes, the experience of chewing and swallowing)
- Wash, shower, or bathe
- Speak with someone (without thinking of what you'll say next or how you'll change the other)
- Answer the phone
- Hug someone
- Cook
- Wash dishes
- Give a baby a bath
- Watch kids sleep
- Notice weather or seasons
- Notice inner weather (what's going on inside emotionally) without judgment

With practice, we eventually become able to respond to any situation with calm awareness.

Integral Yoga: Happy Nature Meditation

Nestled in the beautiful Blue Ridge Mountains of central Virginia, grounds considered sacred by Native Americans, is Yogaville, founded by Sri Swami Satchidananda. Satchidananda (*ananda* means happiness) dedicated his life to teaching people to be happy. There, visitors meditate at 0500 hours for seventy-five minutes—an experience so peaceful and refreshing that they wish it were longer.

This form of meditation is based on his teachings. Like mindfulness, this form of mediation derives from Eastern practices, yet is harmonious with nearly all persuasions.

Sincere and good-humored, Satchidananda taught that happiness is what everyone wants—the criminal, the police officer who chases the criminal, you and I. Happiness comes not from chasing things, but from experiencing our true happy nature and from being useful to others. This meditation focuses on experiencing our true happy nature.

A few points of preparatory instruction: Recall that the purpose of meditation is to experience our true happy nature. This meditation will use three kinds of breathing and mantras, whose only purpose is to settle the mind so you can meditate. The three kinds of breathing are:

- *Abdominal breathing.* As taught in chapter 3, this breathing is, as it were, filling the abdomen on the in-breath and deflating the abdomen on the out-breath. It is gentle, rhythmic, and smooth. As you breathe normally, keep awareness on the breath inside. Let your breathing be a signal to release external attachments and go within—settling in your true happy nature. As agitated water is allowed to settle, it becomes very clear. Allow your breathing to settle your mind.

- *Bellows breathing* presumably expels toxins. Many who are traumatized, anxious, or depressed carry negative emotions in their solar plexus, a mass of nerve cells in the upper abdomen. It is thought that bellows breathing releases these emotions, and perhaps physical wastes, as well. This type of breathing is done by inwardly snapping (contracting) the abdominal muscles. This causes air to be expelled from the lungs. When those muscles are then allowed to fully relax, the lungs naturally fill with air. After the lungs fully inflate, again snap the abdominal muscles. Then relax to inhale. This process is repeated, preparing us to relax and rest in the wisdom mind.

- *Alternate nostril breathing.* The brain follows an ultradian rhythm, whereby dominance shifts every ninety minutes between the right and left hemispheres. Whichever nostril is open tells you which hemisphere is dominant (e.g., if the right nostril is open the left hemisphere is dominant). Alternative nostril breathing is thought to balance the left (logical, linear, externally focused) and right (intuitive, creative, internally focused) hemispheres. This type of breathing is done as follows:
  1. Extend the thumb and ring and little fingers of the right hand. The index and middle fingers are curled and rest in the palm of the hand. Place the thumb against the right side of your nose and the ring and little fingers against the left side of your nose.
  2. Close the right nostril by pressing your thumb against the right side of your nose. Breathe in through the left nostril.
  3. Close the left nostril with your ring and little fingers. Exhale and then inhale through the right nostril.
  4. Close the right nostril then exhale and inhale through the left nostril.
  5. Repeat this cycle of exhaling then inhaling through alternate nostrils.

Practice these three types of breaths until you can do them without looking at the instructions.

A mantra is a word or phrase that is chanted. Mantras have a curiously calming affect. Their effect is not based so much on what the words mean, as on the change in the body and mind that they cause. Focusing on a mantra keeps the focus off of negative thoughts and emotions and helps us to settle into the wisdom mind. In my experience, most people in the West quickly adapt to their use. The three mantras that are chanted in this meditation are:

- *Om* (rhymes with *home*). This mantra denotes peace, oneness within, and oneness with all that is without. Some describe the word as the basic, divine vibration—the sound of God humming or awaking; the primary vibration in the universe heard in the wind, waves, or the hum of an electrical transformer or anything else with power. Chanting the ...*mmmmm* portion of this mantra creates a pleasant vibration in the forehead region, or the area of the prefrontal cortex.

- *Hari Om* (Hah-dee Om). This combination of sounds brings awareness from the stomach, to the thyroid, and then to the top of the head with each successive syllable. This chant helps to ground us in the body and wisdom mind.
- *Shanti Om* (Shahn-tee Om). *Shanti* signifies inner peace. The phrase tends to release tension and suggests lightness.

Practice these mantras until they can be chanted comfortably and naturally. See what happens when you vary the pitch of different syllables, different words within a phrase, or the entire phrase. (Some might choose to use mantras, such as *one* or *love*, instead.)

Some points about meditation are useful to emphasize. There are thousands of methods to meditate—or experience our true happy nature. The breathing and mantras are simply invitations to release attachments and rest in the wisdom mind. The true happy nature is drama-less. Don't expect fireworks when you meditate. It is more likely that your experience will be quiet, pleasant, and subtle. The instructions for Happy Nature Meditation follow. This adaptation takes about thirty minutes. It is practiced once or twice daily. Try it for about a week to see if you'd like to continue it. The times for each step are merely suggestions.

1. Sit quietly in the meditator's posture, like a dignified and steadfast mountain. Relax the muscles of your body. Adopt a light and friendly, almost playful attitude. Imagine that you have just returned from working in the yard. Pleasantly tired, you have nothing left to do or worry about, so you imagine that you sink into a soft chair. When you are ready, gently close your eyes. Use your abdominal breathing as a signal to settle your mind. Just as agitated water becomes clear as it settles, let your mind settle and clear. Breathe abdominally for about five minutes. Release strivings and graspings, content to simply be—resting in your wisdom mind.
2. Chant for a few minutes. Repeat *Om* aloud for about a minute, pausing to allow your mind to settle between repetitions of the word. Repeat this with *Hari Om* and *Shanti Om*.
3. Do bellows breathing for about a minute. Follow this with a minute of abdominal breathing. Repeat this sequence.
4. Do about three minutes of alternate nostril breathing. Notice the pleasant changes in the forehead region.
5. Chant for about a minute, using any combination of Om, Hari Om, and/or Shanti Om. Let the chants settle your mind more.
6. Silently meditate. For about fifteen minutes, release, rest, and relax into your true happy nature. Should thoughts intrude, just greet them cordially and let them pass through awareness like a cloud floating across the sky, as you return your focus to resting in your true happy nature.
7. End with:
    - A minute of chanting, using any combination of Om, Hari Om, and Shanti Om.
    - A minute of intentional chants:
        - "May I be happy & free of suffering."
        - "May I be whole."
        - "May all people be happy & free of suffering."
        - "May all people be whole."
        - "May we all be content."

Before step 7, you might do a smile meditation, letting happiness spread from the face, to the forehead, and to all other parts of the body in sequence. This adds but a few additional minutes.

Resources

Military/Veterans Services

- **Military OneSource** (Tel: 800-342-9647, www.militaryonesource.com). For active duty, Guard, and Reserve members and families. Get a real voice, usually a licensed counselor, 24 hours a day. Initial assessment, then refers to private practice paid for by DOD, up to six sessions. Then referred to Tricare for additional sessions. Also resources for crisis, deployment, injury, and more.

- **Veterans Affairs Facilities.** The U.S. Department of Veterans Affairs (DVA) is the acknowledged expert in treating war-related trauma. DVA offers various treatment options. For compensation, educational, housing, medical, job training or other benefits for PTSD, call or write your local DVA facility (e.g., vet center, regional office). If unable to locate one, call **Department of Veterans Affairs**, Washington, DC (Tel: 800-827-1000; www.va.gov —also check here for veterans service organizations, which can help you find needed help). Vet center readjustment counseling services are available to you if you have served in any combat zone or are a family member of a warrior. You need not be enrolled in the VA. Find a vet center at www.vetcenter.va.gov.

- **Outreach Center of the Defense Centers of Excellence for Psychological Health and TBI** (DCoE) (www.dcoe.health.mil/; Toll free line 866-966-1020) is staffed 24/7 to help anyone find psychological or brain injury resources in your area.

- **www.realwarriors.net.** Maintained by DCoE to build resilience, facilitate recovery, and support reintegration of returning service members, veterans, and their families. Much useful information and links to many resources. Inspiring stories of real service members.

- **The National Center for Telehealth and Technology** (T2) (www.t2health.org/). As the primary DOD office for cutting-edge approaches to the use of technology in the area of psychological health and traumatic brain injury, T2 promotes resilience, recovery, and reintegration of warriors and their families. Its site has a virtual PTSD experience to help service/family members learn about PTSD anonymously, as well as many other excellent resources that you can download or read/listen directly to on your computer. It is also developing free mobile technology apps for smart phones and other portable devices on PTSD, TBI, and/or relaxation/stress management. Search the website, Google *T2 mobile apps*, or search iPhone's AppStore or Android's market place to find out what's available.

- **www.afterdloyment.org.** Wellness resources for the military community include assessments, workshops, videos, and related resources on a broad range of relevant topics.

Books For Warriors Especially

- Grossman, D. *On Combat: The Psychology and Physiology of Deadly Conflict in War and in Peace.* Millstadt, IL: PPCT Research Publications. A very thoughtful work on knowing what to expect and how to prepare to kill when that is required. Lt. Col. Grossman's *On Killing* is also recommended.

- Tick, E. *War and the Soul: Healing Our Nation's Veterans from Post-Traumatic Stress Disorder.* Wheaton, IL: Quest. Tick argues that PTSD is best understood as an identity disorder and soul wound, and moral pain is a root cause. How the honorable warrior soul is healed and reclaimed.

- Hoge, C. W. (2010). *Once A Warrior Always a Warrior: Navigating the Transition from Combat to Home.* Guilford, CT: GPP Life. Covers PTSD, combat stress and mild brain injury/concussions. Practical guidance for many homecoming issues.

PTSD

- Schiraldi, G. R. *The Post-Traumatic Stress Disorder Source Book: A Guide to Healing, Recovery and Growth.* New York: McGraw-Hill. Clearly explains and normalizes the symptoms of PTSD, explains the range of treatment options (e.g., self-managed, professional, groups) and how to find them, and provides a comprehensive listing of resources. "The most valuable, user-friendly manual on PTSD I have ever seen. Must reading for victims, their families, and their therapists." (Dr. George Everly, Executive Editor, *International Journal of Emergency Mental Health*).

Finding a Trauma Specialist
- **SIDRAN Institute**, Baltimore, MD. [Tel: 410-825-8888; help@sidran.org; www.sidran.org]. Helps locate psychotherapists specializing in PTSD. Readings, and other resources.
- **Intensive Trauma Therapy, Inc.**, Morgantown, WV (Tel. 304-291-2912; www.traumatherapy.us). Skillfully combines hypnosis, video technology, and art therapy into 1-2 week intensives with excellent results. Useful for those who wish to shorten their treatment duration. Also trains providers.
- **Anxiety Disorders Association of America**, Silver Spring, MD (Tel: 240-485-1001; www.adaa.org). Provides members with a list of professionals who specialize in the treatment of anxiety disorders. Also provides information on self-help and support groups in your area. Has a catalog of available brochures, books, and audiocassettes. Newsletter. Annual national conference.
- **Mental Health America** (National Mental Health Association), Alexandria, VA (Tel: 703-684-7722; 800-969-NMHA; www.NMHA.org). Provides list of affiliate mental health organizations in your area that can provide resources and information about self-help groups, treatment professionals, and community clinics. Crisis line 1-800-273-TALK.
- **EMDR Institute**, Watsonville, CA (831-761-1040; inst@emdr.com; www.emdr.com). Finding clinicians trained in Eye Movement Densensitization and Reprocessing.
- **Seeking Safety**. To view research and locate Seeking Safety treatment for dual diagnosis of PTSD and substance abuse go to www.seekingsafety.org.

Organizations
- **Rivers of Recovery** [Tel: 303-801-8022; www.riversofrecovery.org] a non-profit outdoor recreational/ rehabilitation program for physically and psychologically injured veterans and active duty military service members and their families.
- **Outward Bound** (Tel: 888-837-5210; www.outwardboundwilderness.org/groups.html). A range of challenging wilderness environments coupled with emotional support to inspire self-respect and care for others, community and environment. Since 1941. Groups customized for survivors of violence, war, sexual assault, incest, cancer, substance use disorders, mild traumatic brain injury, and grief.
- **National Suicide Prevention Lifeline** 800-273-TALK (8255). Immediate assistance for yourself or a loved one you are concerned about.
- **National Domestic Violence Hotline** 800-799-SAFE (7233). Immediate assistance for yourself or a loved one you are concerned about.
- **www.warriorsguidetoinsanity.com** Maintained by a former Marine. Provides help and insights for warriors and their families.

General Resilience Readings
- Ashe, A., & Rampersad, A. *Days of Grace*. New York: Random House. Retaining inner peace and optimism, despite tragedy. By the dignified tennis champion who contracted AIDS from open-heart surgery.
- Frankl, V. *Man's Search for Meaning*. Boston: Beacon. The classic work on discovering meaning in one's life out of suffering. Written by the renowned Holocaust survivor.
- Geisel, Theodor. *Oh, the Places You'll Go*. New York: Random House. Part of the Dr. Seuss series; a clever, humorous treatise on human growth and fallibility.
- Gonzales, L. *Deep Survival: Who Lives, Who Dies, & Why*. New York: Norton. Survival skills that transfer to everyday life include surrender to the situation, reasoned action, calmly take responsibility, and persistence.

- Marx, J. *Season of Life*. New York: Simon & Schuster. Inspired by Viktor Frankl, former NFL star Joe Ehrmann now teaches highly successful young athletes that manhood is not found in athletic prowess, sexual exploitation, and materialism, but in love and meaning.
- McCain, J., with M. Salter. *Why Courage Matters*. New York: Random House. As Mother Teresa noted, everything lies in having courage for whatever comes in life. Provocative insights rooting courage in love.
- Opdyke, I.G. *In My Hands*. New York: Anchor. Stirring story of the courageous Holocaust rescuer who remained tender inside, despite incalculable suffering.
- Schiraldi, G. R. *The Complete Guide to Resilience: Why It Matters, How to Build and Maintain It*. Ashburn, VA: Resilience Training International. The clear and comprehensive guide for everyone, in any role or station in life.
- Schiraldi, G. R. *World War II Survivors: Lessons in Resilience*. Ellicott City, MD: Chevron. Forty-one combat survivors explain how they preserved their sanity and the ability to function under many forms of extreme duress. Their lessons are applicable to all of us today.
- Schiraldi, G. R. *The Self-Esteem Workbook*. Oakland, CA: New Harbinger. Based on the successful "Stress and the Healthy Mind" course, University of Maryland. Detailed instructions for many effective skills.
- Schiraldi, G. R. *Ten Simple Solutions for Building Self-Esteem*. Oakland, CA: New Harbinger. Combines cognitive behavioral, mindfulness, and ACT strategies. Based on the effective "Beyond 9/11: Stress, Survival, and Coping" course, University of Maryland.
- Schiraldi, G.R., & Kerr, M.H. *The Anger Management Sourcebook*. New York: McGraw-Hill. "A must for those who are serious about managing their anger more effectively." (R. J. Hedaya, M.D., Clinical Professor of Psychiatry, Georgetown University Hospital).
- Schiraldi, G. R. *Conquer Anxiety, Worry and Nervous Fatigue: A Guide to Greater Peace*. Ellicott City, MD: Chevron. From hyperventilation to worrisome thoughts. "The best book for anxiety we've ever seen" (Sidran Institute).

Couples and Family Skills
- Markman, H., Stanley, S., & Blumberg, S. L. *Fighting <u>for</u> Your Marriage: Positive Steps for Preventing Divorce and Preserving a Lasting Love*. San Francisco: Jossey-Bass. From conflict resolution to increasing fun. Practical. Based on solid research.
- Prevention and Relationship Enhancement Program: Resources for a Loving Relationship, Denver, Colorado (Tel: 800-366-0166). *Fighting <u>for</u> Your Marriage* and other books. Four excellent, inexpensive, practical DVDs to help develop communication skills, solve problems, and promote intimacy. The PREP program is well researched and respected.
- Lundberg, G., & Lundberg, J. *I Don't Have to Make Everything All Better*. New York: Viking Penguin. Treasure chest of methods for relating to people. Learn how to walk alongside people emotionally (validating), rather than arguing or criticizing.
- Lundberg, G., & Lundberg, J. *Married for Better, Not Worse: The Fourteen Secrets to a Happy Marriage*. Another down-to-earth treasure for creating a satisfying marriage.
- Latham, G. I. *The Power of Positive Parenting: A Wonderful Way to Raise Children*. No. Logan, UT: P&T ink. Useful and thorough guide to steady, consistent, and peaceful parenting.
- Garcia-Prats, C. M., & Garcia-Prats, J. A. *Good Families Don't Just Happen: What We Learned From Raising Our Ten Sons and How It Can Work For You*. Holbrook, MA: Adams Media Corporation. Principle-based skills, starting with respect between spouses.
- www.foreverfamilies.net. For those who prefer to work off the web, this has been found to work as well as workshops. Instructions for many exercises on all aspects of strengthening marriage and family. Spiritual bent, but anyone can apply the useful skills independent of orientation.
- All Family Resources (www.familymanagement.com). Rich range of topics from parenting to dealing with crisis.

Physical Fitness

- *Flow Motion: The Simplified T'ai Chi Workout.* DVD by C. J. McPhee & D. Ross. Los Angeles: Lightworks Audio & Video. Gentle beginner's workouts in tai chi, which has been found to lower blood pressure and improve fitness.
- Christensen, A. *Easy Does It Yoga.* New York: Fireside. Instructions for gentle postures for the aged, injured, or inactive. Many can be done desk-side to relax and increase energy and flexibility, and are thus useful for all.

Nutrition

- USDA's www.MyPyramind.gov helps you make an eating plan that is tailored to your needs. Based on solid research, this user-friendly site offers a wealth of useful information.
- A user-friendly website to count calories in everyday and restaurant/fast foods is http://nutritiondata.com.
- DASH diet Plan at www.nhlbi.nih.gov/health/public/heart/hbp/dash. Free to view, nominal charge for hard copy. The DASH eating plan has been found to improve cardiovascular health.

Heart Coherence

- **Institute of HeartMath**, Boulder Creek, CA   (Tel: 800-711-6221; email info@heartmath.com; www.heartmath.org; www.Heartmathstore.com). Contact for books, videos, music, and other products related to heart coherence, as well as to purchase emWave products that enables one to monitor heart rhythms in real time as one practices HeartMath skills.
- **StressEraser.** This portable device uses the breath to increase heart coherence (Tel: 760-448-5588; http://stresseraser.com).

Happiness Books

- Brooks, A. C. *Gross National Happiness: Why Happiness Matters for America – and How We Can Get More of It.* New York: Basic. An accomplished researcher draws upon large and reputable data bases, mostly from recent studies, to draw conclusions on topics ranging from politics, family, and religious values as they relate to happiness.
- Lyubomirsky, S. *The How of Happiness: A Scientific Approach to Getting the Life You Want.* New York: Penguin. A masterful combination of solid research and practical, tested methods to enhance happiness.

Mindfulness

Mindfulness-Based Stress Reduction (MBSR)

- Search mindfulness or mindfulness-based stress reduction for local resources.
- University of Massachusetts Medical Center, Center for Mindfulness (www.umassmed.edu) hosts training and identifies places where MBSR classes are available.
- Mindfulness meditation CDs and tapes by Jon Kabat-Zinn, Ph.D. (www.stressreductiontapes.com).

Mindfulness Books

- Schiraldi, G. R. *Ten Simple Solutions for Building Self-Esteem.* Oakland, CA: New Harbinger. Includes instructions for mindfulness meditation within the context of self-esteem enhancement.
- Kabat-Zinn, J. *Full Catastrophe Living.* New York: Bantam Dell. Still the classic work.
- Brach, T. *Radical Acceptance: Embracing your Life with the Heart of a Buddha.* New York: Bantam.
- Brantley, J. *Calming Your Anxious Mind: How Mindfulness and Compassion Can Free You From Anxiety, Fear, and Panic.* Oakland, CA: New Harbinger.

Notes

www.ingramcontent.com/pod-product-compliance
Lightning Source LLC
Chambersburg PA
CBHW080522090426
42734CB00015B/3132